D1503445

THE HEALTHCARE CUSTOMER SERVICE REVOLUTION

The Growing Impact of Managed Care on Patient Satisfaction

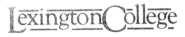

310 S. Peoria St. Ste. 512
Chicago, Il 60607 3534

Phone 312-226-6294
Fax 312-226-6405

THE HEALTHCARE CUSTOMER SERVICE REVOLUTION

The Growing Impact of Managed Care on Patient Satisfaction

DAVID ZIMMERMAN

PEGGY ZIMMERMAN

CHARLES LUND

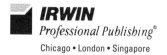

IRWIN
Professional Publishing®
Chicago • London • Singapore

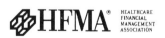

HFMA® HEALTHCARE
FINANCIAL
MANAGEMENT
ASSOCIATION

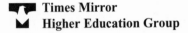 **Times Mirror**
Higher Education Group

Library of Congress Cataloging-in-Publication Data

Zimmerman, David R.
   The healthcare customer service revolution: the growing impact of
managed care on patient satisfaction / David Zimmerman,
Peggy Zimmerman, Charles Lund.
     p.   cm.
  Includes index.
  ISBN 0–7863–0893–1
  1. Patient satisfaction. 2. Medical personnel and patient.
3. Medical care—Quality control. 4. Hospitals—Administration—
—Case studies. I. Zimmerman, Peggy. II. Lund, Charles. III. Title.
R727.3.Z56 1996
362.1'068—dc20   95–43460

Printed in the United States of America
1 2 3 4 5 6 7 8 9 0 BS 2 1 0 9 8 7 6 5

*To the memory of our loving father,
Carl Lund, a jovial man who always made
us feel so worthwhile in spite of our own
shortcomings and failures.*

PREFACE

The Healthcare Customer Service Revolution is an outgrowth from the experiences that we have seen first-hand through our professional assignments and experienced personally as patients, wives, husbands, parents, daughters, and sons.

We have surveyed thousands of patients and interviewed dozens of employers throughout the country to get their reactions to their personal experiences in healthcare situations. They all confirm that what needs to be improved in the healthcare arena is the human element.

The fact is that most people in healthcare entered their profession to give something back—they had a driving need to help humanity and make a difference, but somewhere they became disconnected. We need to shed that superiority complex and rediscover that keen desire to work for a noble goal and get back to the basics of human dignity.

As a mother of a large family, I have the opportunity to get into hospitals, doctors' offices, and clinics on a regular basis. Although my experiences at many of them have been positive, I can almost always cite problems relating to customer service. Rarely does a healthcare facility treat me as a customer and not just another patient.

Attitude is everything; indifference breeds anger and hostility. The basics of good human relations coupled with excellent medical care can create a special kind of synergy.

People have a great thirst for smiles. They have an enormous longing for cheerfulness and encouragement. Each day we encounter a good number of patients who await that momentary gift of our joy. They are extremely grateful for small acts of human kindness.

Gratitude is a human virtue that adds a great deal to social life. It consists of affectionate recognition when a favor is received. This virtue contributes remarkably to a more friendly environment.

Throughout the course of our professional work we should sense the importance of friendship, cordiality, temperance, love for the truth, understanding, loyalty, optimism, and sincerity. These social virtues make daily life more pleasant. In my opinion, these are the critical ingredients that are missing in an otherwise exceptional healthcare system in this country.

Our incomprehensible advances in medicine have given the medical profession the "Midas touch." What is needed now is the "human touch."

Peggy Zimmerman

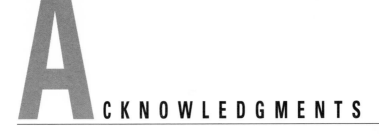

Acknowledgments

Our thanks to those who spent many hours to assist us in this project: Sandee Klopfer, Tim Malaney, Chris Mroz, Bruce Nelson, Elizabeth Ridley, Christy Zimmerman, and Mike Zimmerman. Our gratitude to the many who shared their personal experiences as patients in our nation's healthcare providers. Finally, to those hospitals that allowed us to learn from them what successful customer service can mean to the public, we are extremely grateful.

CONTENTS

3 CHAPTER

Managed Care's Monetary Measures   27

4 CHAPTER

Competing Means Satisfying Patients   41

5 CHAPTER

6 CHAPTER

7 CHAPTER

8 CHAPTER

9 CHAPTER

Unleashing Customer Service through Servant Leadership 117

10 CHAPTER

Focus on Customer Service 135

11 CHAPTER

12 CHAPTER

13 CHAPTER

14 CHAPTER

An "Aloha" Approach to Patient Relations: The Queen's Medical Center   183

15 CHAPTER

Customer Service Commandos: Holy Cross Hospital's War to Improve Patient Satisfaction   195

1

CHAPTER

The Revolution
Has Begun

A physician was recently confronted by a 40-year-old female patient detailing the mistakes that the physician's office staff had made. The doctor responded, "Well, you can go somewhere else if you want to." This scenario exemplifies the attitudes of many healthcare providers regarding customer service.

When we asked this patient what aspects of customer service from a healthcare provider were important to her, she answered, "I expect them to see me as a person . . . that they use my name, look at me, and show a certain amount of empathy. I also expect a sense of personal service regarding the bills and the reduction in long delay times." These are certainly not unrealistic expectations for patients to have from their healthcare provider. However, patients say their expectations are not being met.

The revolution for improved customer service by healthcare providers has begun. For years, Americans have told opinion pollsters that they felt disenchanted, disenfranchised, and alienated from healthcare providers. Every available study indicates that patients no longer view providers as angels of mercy.

Until recently, patients had no formal mechanism to voice displeasure with the way they were treated by the apathetic hospital staff or the pious, egocentric physician and his cold, indifferent staff. Managed care, which is rapidly taking over the industry, is changing all of that. Now patients are being asked by HMOs and PPOs to score their hospitals and physicians on customer service issues. Employers and managed care organizations are evaluating patient feedback and taking action.

Within the past several years, the nation's employers have gained control of the way healthcare is delivered in this country. Their choice of controlling the delivery system is primarily through the managed care concept. During the 1990s, controlling health costs has been the major objective of employers. In fact, in 1994, the average healthcare cost per employee actually dropped slightly. The 1.1 percent decrease U.S. employers realized in 1994 reflected the first decline in healthcare costs in 20 years. Justifiably, employers feel they have begun to control their healthcare costs and are now turning their attention to quality of care. Under the heading of "quality of care" falls customer service or patient satisfaction.

For instance, in the summer of 1995, a group of representatives of some of the country's largest employers and purchasers of health insurance agreed to pursue a fundamental shift in emphasis in the nation's managed healthcare systems: Now that costs have begun to be controlled, they want the primary focus to be placed on measuring the quality of care. The broad-based agreement was reached at Jackson Hole, Wyoming, by 30 officials of federal, state, and local public employees' organizations, consumer groups, and officials of such major employers as American Express, the Minnesota Mining and Manufacturing Company, the

Ameritech Corporation, and Pepsico. All together they represented an estimated 80 million consumers of health insurance.

"Monitoring quality will be the next battlefield," said Tom J. Elkin, assistant executive director of the California Public Employees Retirement System, which represents more than 800,000 state and local government employees and their families. He predicted that only health plans and providers that demonstrate high quality would still be in existence by the year 2000. Two elements of the consensus that emerged were regarded as significant by leaders in healthcare. One was that purchasers of healthcare for such large numbers of consumers with great potential power in the marketplace were united in their desire for greater attention to quality. The second was a decision to put into motion a plan to gather data in a more uniform and comprehensive way than ever before on the medical outcomes for various methods of treating patients for major illnesses.[1]

More employees are now grouped together through managed care companies than ever before. Those employees who become patients now have a unified voice and their perceptions of their healthcare are being heard. Employees now have a method of expression. More important, the employers care about what their employees think about their healthcare service. How patients are treated as human beings is now becoming an issue the employer tracks, evaluates, trends, and communicates to the managed care companies and providers.

CUSTOMER SERVICE WILL IMPACT REVENUE

Customer service, long given a low priority by providers, now becomes so important that it can affect their cash flow and revenue. Employers are saying to providers and managed care companies, "Score well in customer service or

---

1. *The New York Times,* July 5, 1995.

you'll get your knuckles wrapped, you'll be scolded, or worse yet, your bonus will be stripped, or you'll lose our patients altogether." Providers who flunk the customer service test will lose patients. It won't be a few disgruntled patients who take their business somewhere else because of the poor service they received from the provider—it will be large numbers of patients taken away through the managed care network. They will turn to the provider who knows what customer service is all about and can provide it successfully.

Customer service has indeed become the new battlefield for providers in this day of the new paradigm in healthcare delivery. Cost control and excellent customer service will go hand-in-hand. Employers with newfound leverage in healthcare will make certain it happens. And make no mistake about it: Patients and their families are the customers for providers. Customers are no longer the medical staff, or payers for hospitals, or the payers for physicians, but the people receiving the care or their relatives.

When the three of us decided to write this book, we put together a research plan in early 1995 that called for personally interviewing a large number of Fortune 500 companies and a good sampling of managed care companies. The objective was to learn their attitude and approach toward customer service of providers to their employees and subscribers. We wanted to learn whether providers' customer service was important enough for them to track and evaluate and what they would do with the data once collected. If they did track that aspect of healthcare delivery, what would they do about the providers who did not score well?

During the summer months of 1995, we personally interviewed more than 25 large employers representing millions of employees in locations all across the country. Included were: Boeing, Borden, Coca-Cola, First Chicago Bank, General Electric, Hallmark Cards, Hershey Foods, Hewlett-Packard, Johnson Wax, Kellogg's, Kimberly-Clark,

Marriott Corp., McDonald's, Nike, Inc., J. C. Penney, Procter & Gamble, Sara Lee, Sherwin-Williams, Time-Warner, Toys 'R' Us, UPS, Walgreen's, Walt Disney Co., Warner-Lambert, and Wrigley Co. Nearly half of these corporations ranked in the top 100 most-admired companies in *Fortune* magazine's recent listing of "America's Most Admired Corporations."[2] These companies will set the pace for the rest of America's employers in demanding improved patient satisfaction and customer service from the nation's healthcare providers.

We also conducted personal telephone interviews with large- and mid-sized managed care companies representing more than 25 million enrollees, to determine their approach to tracking and evaluating customer service at the provider level. Included in the interviews with managed care organizations were the following: Kaiser Permanente, Beech Street of California, Health Service Network, Preferred Care, ConnectiCare, Medica Primary, The Prudential, Virginia Health Network, FHP of Colorado, Humana, Cigna, American Lifecare, Choice Care, IHC, and King Co. Medical.

We also conducted interviews with nearly 50 hospitals to determine their approach toward customer service. We made on-site visits to a half dozen of those hospitals in order to obtain a better feel for their customer service approach. Some of interviews lasted a day or two; others covered a week or more. We were attempting to discover specifically what facilities were doing to improve their patient relations and what their future customer service plans might include. We also asked the hospitals and medical groups what they thought were the most important factors in excellent patient relations; how they tracked customer satisfaction; and *who* (in their opinion) is the customer: community employers? payers? their medical staff? the patients and their families?

---

2. *Fortune,* March 1995.

PATIENT DISSATISFACTION WITH CUSTOMER SERVICE BY HOSPITALS AND PHYSICIANS

We also wanted a good sense for what the patient thought about customer service at the provider level in healthcare. We conducted written, mailback surveys with former patients (patients within the last six months from the date of service), as well as hundreds of personal interviews with former patients. The patient interviews and survey included nearly 2,000 people in 17 states who had received care from 30 different hospitals and hundreds of physicians' offices within the last year. Our investigation also included in-depth discussions with such well-known patient survey organizations as Press-Ganey, Healthcare Research Systems, and The Picker Foundation.

The hundreds of hours of interviews and painstaking research led us to the observations you will find in the succeeding chapters. We feel it is the most up-to-date look at the organized patient revolt against poor customer service by healthcare providers and at the growing trend of the employer to tie cash to customer satisfaction. The revolutionary trends we uncovered revealed that employers are placing a higher emphasis on employee/patient satisfaction than ever before and that patients are fed up with indifferent, cold, uncaring service they receive from hospitals and physician offices. The employers and patient both want a change and they will get it.

We found nearly 60 percent of the Fortune 500 employers we interviewed presently survey and track employee satisfaction for provider customer service issues; another 21 percent of them told us they plan to start tracking soon. That means nearly 80 percent of the nation's largest employers will be tracking customer service issues. Nearly 100 percent of the managed care companies said they survey and monitor provider patient satisfaction with their enrollees. Over 50 percent of the employers and managed care companies said they will drop providers who flunk the customer service standards they set. In fact, some have switched providers already for that very reason: poor customer service.

Our surveys and interviews of more than 2,000 former patients showed they are not satisfied with customer service in hospitals or medical offices. Although 90 percent of those surveyed said customer service was *extremely* important to them, they reported that both their hospital and doctor fell far short of their expectations. On a 10-point satisfaction index, hospitals scored a low 7.4 and their physicians only slightly better at 8.1. These findings of ours coincided with the results of a University of Michigan research project designed to measure the quality of American goals and services. That study of 46,000 customers scored hospitals only a 74 on a 100-point satisfaction index—just above the postal service and just behind long distance telephone services.[3]

Amazingly, our survey revealed that 6 percent of the patients who responded said the customer service aspect was so bad they would not return to that hospital, and 8 percent said they would tell the world how badly they were treated so others would not be faced with the same "poor service and humiliation." "Lack of human respect," was a complaint they often reiterated. Patients told us that they defined good customer service by the provider as good old-fashioned actions such as communicating with them, showing compassion, fast service, and (the old stand-by) friendliness. There were no surprises there; certainly such actions are not difficult to provide. However, patients reported in no uncertain terms it's not happening nearly often enough.

---

3. *Modern Healthcare,* December 19–26, 1994, p. 38. This and all similar subsequent references are reprinted with permission from Modern Healthcare, copyright Crain Communications, Inc., 740 N. Rush St., Chicago, IL 60611.

We asked former patients to describe the term *customer service;* following are some of the responses:

Fast and friendly check in and out; compassionate and friendly treatments from nurses and doctors.

Adequate parking; wheelchair availability at the door; prompt, courteous, and cheerful customer relations.

Courteous and helpful. "In tune" with patients' needs.

Registration and admittance without long delays and with courtesy.

Being taken care of and having questions answered in a quick, friendly manner.

Answering questions, giving information, showing directions, making people understand.

Courteous treatment by personnel. It is important to make their patient feel that she is important and her needs will be met.

Having the staff listen to your questions or complaints and also discussing your bill later. I guess I equate "customer service" with communications.

HOSPITALS' APPROACH TO CUSTOMER SERVICE SHOWS LITTLE INGENUITY

We also spoke with nearly 50 hospitals having bed sizes ranging from 46 to 949 in various geographical regions regarding their approach toward improved patient satisfaction. Most of what we found has been going on in the industry for years. Almost every hospital has some kind of a patient survey or questionnaire to determine how patients felt about the customer service aspect of their visit. About one-third of the hospitals we talked to use an outside firm such as Press-Ganey to conduct the patient survey and report the findings. The rest have their own in-house patient survey process.

Nearly one-third of the hospitals said they had some kind of customer service training program for their employees. Again, such programs have been fairly common practice for years. The other most common practices we uncovered were focus groups (16 percent), specific process changes to cut waiting time (16 percent), patient-focused care reengineering or restructuring (14 percent), development of a special department (usually called the patient representative department) (16 percent), formation of a special committee or task force (9 percent), and development of specific standards of customer service excellence (9 percent).

Most experts interviewed by *Modern Healthcare* magazine last year didn't think hospitals were serious enough about improving customer satisfaction. However, an increasing number are starting to document satisfaction for payers, employers, and the public out of fear they will lose patients and revenue. Industry leaders in customer satisfaction, such as the Marriott Corp., are far ahead of hospitals in developing programs to reward employees for treating their customers well, experts told *Modern Healthcare*.[4]

Although the vast majority of hospitals said the patient or family was their customer, another 63 percent told us their medical staff was also their customer, another 50 percent said the payers were also their customer, and 22 percent told us their community employers were also considered their customer. In our opinion, this may be part of the problem for providers in their attempt to focus on improved customer relations. Because of their confusion about who their target of service really is and trying to be all things to all people, they fail altogether in many in-

4. *Modern Healthcare,* July 18, 1994, p. 30.

stances. When we asked each hospital its plans for the future regarding upgrading their customer service, we generally got more of what the facility is already doing with a few exceptions.

Providers will have to face up to the negative image many Americans have of their healthcare service, then do something about it. This includes every area of human contact within every healthcare institution in the country. Hospitals and medical groups can no longer compete on the strength of their clinical expertise alone because the industry is having to react to competition that can and will provide the care for less cost. What sets providers apart today is the success of their "service" efforts.

More and more, the service and patient relations context that surrounds the medical care given will give providers added value and will differentiate them from the competition. Patients are up in arms, believing that they are treated with a lack of dignity, respect, and compassion. They are mad, and now that they can voice their displeasure, their anger will hit providers at the bottom line. Future business in the form of patient volume will swing in the balance, based a great deal on provider customer service.

It's a new battlefield that providers themselves have created by their apathy toward customer service. Dissatisfaction has been festering in patients' minds for a long time, fueling the revolt for improved customer service. And today patients are leading it.

2

Customer Service

The Next Battleground

Since the mid-1980s, dramatic changes have occurred in the healthcare delivery system. The concept of managed care is rapidly taking control of the industry. Ten years ago, 15 million Americans were enrolled in health maintenance organizations (HMOs). That number skyrocketed to 47.2 million as of July 1994, according to a report by *Interstudy*. More than 100 million Americans are enrolled in HMOs or preferred provider organizations (PPOs). Managed care, with its emphasis on controlling treatment and containing costs, is changing the way healthcare services are delivered. Gone forever are the simpler days of fee-for-service healthcare. Today's managed care world of medicine is more complex, and ultimately more controversial, than anything that has gone before.

The vast majority of people who participate in managed care programs are enrolled through their workplace, which means that the employers themselves have been

suddenly and dramatically thrust into the role of interme-
diary in the formerly sacrosanct provider/patient relationship. As a result, the employer has gained the leverage of
control from the providers and payers. "We've had a revolution in this country in terms of the accountability of
healthcare purchasers," says Helen Darling, manager of
healthcare strategy and programs for Xerox Corp. "There's
been a paradigm shift in terms of who's in charge that
began in the early 1980s."

"The biggest news story missed in the last decade has
been business' impact on healthcare," echoes David
Langness, vice president of the Healthcare Association of
Southern California. "Employers have had the largest impact
on healthcare costs—not physicians, hospitals, or health
plans."[1] Large employers represent huge patient bases.
Managed care companies are feeling that pressure, and as
a result have recognized the need to woo, win, and keep the
contracts of large, powerful employers. The best way to do
that, of course, is for the managed care companies to make
sure that their subscribers—the employers' employees—
are satisfied with their healthcare experiences.

Managed care offers the potential patient fewer choices
in terms of the who, what, when, where, and why of seeking
medical treatment. In exchange, it promises lower premiums, caps on out-of-pocket expenses, and potentially better
service. But better service as judged by whose standards?
Employers expect efficiency and quality from their providers, and are beginning now to demand statistical evidence
to prove that their healthcare choices are meeting the needs
and desires of their employees. This statistical evidence
comes from two primary sources: the surveys done by a
company overall among its employees, and the survey results provided to the employer by the managed care company. The results illustrate the measured level of satisfaction
among enrollees in a particular HMO or PPO. Regardless

---

1. *Hospitals & Health Networks*, May 5, 1995.

of the source of the information, the bottom line issue is and will continue to be to an even greater extent, *whether the patient is satisfied with the care he or she receives.*

MOST OF THE NATION'S LARGEST EMPLOYERS WILL BE TRACKING CUSTOMER SERVICE BY PROVIDERS

As noted in Chapter 1, nearly 60 percent of the companies we interviewed presently survey their employees to determine the level of their satisfaction with their managed care company and their providers, and another 21 percent stated that they were going to start surveying and tracking their employee satisfaction with providers. Eighty percent of the nation's largest and most progressive employers will be tracking customer service issues.

As hospitals and physicians compete for patients, and employers shop around for the best benefit packages to offer their employees, patient satisfaction and customer service are suddenly major concerns for everyone in both the healthcare industry, and in industry overall. A revolution is underway in the healthcare world: Employees are telling their employers what they want and need in healthcare services, and the employers in turn are pressuring the managed care companies to find providers who measure up.

Nowhere is this equation clearer than at First Chicago Bank in Chicago, Illinois. First Chicago employs 18,500 people, which translates into 18,500 potential HMO enrollees. Robert Bonin, First Chicago's manager of benefits administration, says his company's two HMOs are eager to work with First Chicago on issues related to employee/patient satisfaction. "We are the flagship employer for both of our HMOs," Bonin explains. "It's not a question of how open are they, but how quickly will they do it? I would say they are totally open because the alternative is, I dump them, take my $20 million and give it to someone else," he says. "We've done that. We've canceled our largest network and made our smallest local network our largest local network because we were unable to come to terms. So they [managed care companies] are well-motivated to look at things."

Many major U.S. employers are starting to realize the importance of good customer service in healthcare and have begun to pay more attention to the care and kindness received by their employees as they use healthcare benefits. To many people, it just makes good sense. "The more you move into managed care and the less choice an associate has regarding where he or she goes, it becomes more incumbent upon the employer to be sure that what their choices are, are making them [the employees] at least moderately happy," says Marcia McLeod, manager of benefits program development at J.C. Penney's corporate headquarters in Dallas.

Bill Greer, the director of benefits for Kellogg's Company in Battle Creek, Michigan, agrees. His company recently surveyed one-third of its 7,000 employees about healthcare. "Because we're putting in managed care, we want to track what's going on. We hope to be able to show that our managed care plan is a higher quality than our other plans. We don't know if that will happen or not," he admits.

This sentiment is echoed by Robert Wittcoff, director of employee benefits for McDonald's Corporation in Oak Brook, Illinois. His corporation is also beginning to get more involved with tracking employee/patient satisfaction. "We're a service business and we've learned that, for a business, it's very important to keep our customers happy; and if you take that to the next logical step, you've got to keep employees happy. We're spending gobs of money on healthcare, and it doesn't make sense to spend that money and not have satisfied employees," he says. "Healthcare, whether we like it or not, is becoming part of our business."

QUALITY BECOMES KEY STRATEGY

In addition to keeping their employees happy, companies have a huge financial interest vested in their employees' healthcare. A 1994 survey by Foster Higgins found that total healthcare benefit costs averaged $3,741 per employee per year. The importance of improving the quality of the care received for those precious healthcare dollars is recognized by many corporate executives.

"We wanted to drive quality in terms of healthcare as a very key strategy towards healthcare cost management. We're trying to improve the value for the dollar," says Richard Dreyfuss, director of employee benefits at Hershey Food Corporation in Hershey, Pennsylvania.

"Looking at what you're getting for the dollar is something that I think companies need to focus on more, particularly as it relates to outcome measurement and patient satisfaction," Dreyfuss says. Hershey Foods recently surveyed all 6,500 of its employees with a written questionnaire on healthcare. The company then used the results to help design a better health plan and to work with individual providers to improve their services. "That's valuable data when you walk into someone's office and you try to address a specific issue. There's just no substitute for having facts," he says.

And those facts help Hershey's employees to make better healthcare choices for themselves and their families. Hershey Foods offers its employees choices among four HMOs and its own point-of-service plan. "I think people are more accommodating or more accepting of the managed care way of buying healthcare now. Price is an issue, but I don't think it's as big an issue as everybody thinks it is. They [the employees] may select the most expensive option if that's the way it comes out in terms of their values."

One common concern voiced by employees pushed into managed care by their employers is that such strict attention to cost control on the part of the insurers will automatically translate into a compromise on the quality of the care they receive. Not so, insists Bill Ruoff, leader of insurance benefits delivery for GE headquarters in Schenectady, New York. "One of the things we work really hard at, in terms of our communication with the employees, is to assure them that yes, we are in fact trying to save money, no question about that; on the other hand, saving money doesn't mean that we're going to short-change the quality of the care that you receive. And we have actions, things that we do to back up that claim," Ruoff says.

Employers will force their managed care companies to make customer service a part of the contractual negotiations with providers. For instance, to encourage HMOs to improve customer satisfaction and the quality of their care, a business group negotiated agreements in which the HMO could lose 2 percent of its premiums if it failed to achieve specified improvements in customer satisfaction and quality of care.

A group of large companies in California recently negotiated an average price cut of 4.3 percent in 1996 for their employees' healthcare from a group of 13 HMOs in the state. It was the second consecutive year that companies belonging to the Pacific Business Group on Health have obtained price reductions. For 1996 the HMOs offered contracts that ranged from no price increase to a decline of 13 percent.[2]

Patricia Powers, head of the California business coalition, said 13 of the 15 HMOs working with her group agreed to cut their rates. A major reason, she told *The Wall Street Journal,* is that health plans themselves can negotiate lower prices from providers of medical care. "There's an oversupply of hospitals and physicians."[3] "It's a buyer's marketplace right now," according to Glenn Meister, a Foster Higgins & Co. health-insurance consultant. "As employers head into renewal negotiations for 1996, we're seeing expectations of a zero percent increase, or even a decrease."[4]

---

2. *The New York Times,* June 22, 1995.
3. *The Wall Street Journal,* June 22, 1995.
4. Ibid.

EMPLOYERS BECOME THE PATIENT'S CHAMPION

From an employee/patient standpoint, one of the great advantages of having the employer suddenly so involved in their healthcare decisions is the chance to have a powerful ally on their side when confronting the HMO or PPO. Robert Bonin calls the employer the patient's "champion" in any healthcare debate and offers this illustration from his own experiences at First Chicago:

> We had an employee with a great big lump on his head. HMO member. Cosmetic surgery. How would you like to go walking around with a lump two inches long and an inch and a half wide and about three centimeters thick, on your forehead? That's cosmetic? But it is. Two doctors say it is cosmetic. But don't you think we should use a little judgment here? Without a champion, the system would say no. "Go in peace. Just don't lay on it." So we caused them, I think, to be a little more rational, or patient-oriented in their thinking. Without our focusing on the patient, there would be less focus by the health plan on the patient, believe me.

This added pressure by the employer on obtaining health benefits can manifest itself in several ways. For many companies, it means first surveying employees on healthcare, and then requiring the HMO or PPO to survey its members and provide those results to the company, and to account for any discrepancies. "With our managed care plans, we measure employees both through the company and through the supplier. Most of the managed care plans, as a requirement for contracting with us, are compelled to survey customers on various service-oriented parameters. We make that part and parcel of their job," says Bill Ruoff of GE. "We do that for one of two reasons. To measure something very specific that we're interested in knowing about, or basically, to keep our suppliers honest, to make sure that the feedback we get is correlating with the feedback that they're giving to us."

But most employers are quick to add that in most cases, the managed care company is as concerned about getting accurate information as the employer is. "I made it sound like we bludgeon people, and we're certainly willing to do that if we need to, but I don't think there's going to be a need to bludgeon anybody," says Bonin of First Chicago. "I think that they (managed care companies) are seriously interested in the results and what they may do to improve themselves."

EMPLOYER'S PERSPECTIVE: WHAT DO PATIENTS/ EMPLOYEES REALLY WANT?

So what do healthcare patients want? Care. Compassion. Concern. Those are things so basic providers might just take them for granted. But even the simplest issues like friendliness, cheerfulness, and privacy will become more important as employees rate their healthcare experiences and make their choices for future care. And because these issues are so important to employees, they will be important to employers as well, in the long run.

"There are other ways to measure quality, but certainly it's the more subjective issues that you want to look at, too. Do you feel like you're being treated with respect, in a timely manner, do they feel like they're getting quality care? That's an important piece of it," says Marcia McLeod of J. C. Penney's.

Sensitivity on the part of the provider is an important issue too. "One of our most important concerns is a doctor who shows sensitivity to the employee's needs," says Ronald Kastler, human resources manager for benefits, education, and communication, at Johnson Wax in Racine, Wisconsin. Also important is the doctor's awareness of the patient's "life events."

"A young person with a family has different concerns and healthcare needs than a single person with elderly parents, and a sensitive doctor or hospital staff should be aware of those differences," Kastler says.

The best employers also realize that the job an employee does may affect his or her conception of customer service from the provider. Marcia McLeod of J. C. Penney's recognizes the connection; her employees are required to perform to a high standard of customer service, and they expect the same level of service when they are on the receiving end of care: "Their main job in life is going out and smiling at people and trying to be nice to them and provide customer service. They expect the same from others," she explains.

HOW EMPLOYERS USE THE DATA THEY RECEIVE

Our research has shown that most major U.S. companies do survey their employees, right down to the specific level of satisfaction with individual providers. But what happens to that information once it is gathered? Is it filed away in a locked cabinet, never to see daylight again, or do employers actually use that data?

"They use it," says Melissa Kennedy, vice-president of HealthCare Research Systems, a healthcare surveying and consulting firm at Ohio State University that has performed surveying for several major employers, including Xerox, GE, Digital, and GTE. "People that we talk to in hospitals get these huge reports and they sit on someone's desk for months and months and months. Employers and health plans are dying for this data because they're using it at the negotiations table constantly," she says. "They're using it a lot because when you're on the employer's and the managed care side of things, there's a direct relationship between what can be drawn from these results and the money that can be saved by using these data."

For many employers, the first way the survey results are used is to change the plans themselves according to what employees have indicated they wanted. For example, when many second- and third-shift workers at S. C. Johnson Wax in Racine, Wisconsin, complained on their surveys about no doctors being available during the hours they were off work, Johnson Wax worked with its HMO and arranged for one of the doctors in the plan to reschedule some hours to be available at more unusual times, for example, from 11 AM to 7 PM. The company saw great improvement in the survey results the following year. Here is a clear example of an employer gleaning information from a survey, data not obtainable any other way, then using that information on behalf of the employee. Ask yourself whether the typical American assembly line worker could phone the doctor and persuade him or her to schedule an appointment for 7 PM on a Friday night. But that's precisely what the employer has succeeded in doing.

There are other uses for survey results, too. Kellogg's uses its survey results to target both educational and intervention efforts. The company also uses the data to risk-adjust the company's healthcare costs. At J. C. Penney's, survey information is used as feedback for the managed care plans, so managed care managers know how associates perceive them. The company may also eventually use those survey results for negotiations when it comes time to renew contracts with specific managed care plans and their network of providers. "We plan on using that information for whatever good reasons there are to use it," says Marcia McLeod.

In a slightly different vein, First Chicago Bank publishes the results of its surveys and makes that information available to employees as they decide which plan to join. "I don't know if anybody changed his or her mind based on the information, but the plan that consistently got the highest scores is our biggest plan, and also our least expensive plan. So it had the highest satisfaction, lowest cost, and highest membership," says Robert Bonin.

THE PROBLEM OF LOW-SCORING PROVIDERS: WHAT WILL EMPLOYERS DO?

In worst-case scenarios, doctors and hospitals that score low on patient satisfaction surveys among employees may be dropped from the healthcare network at the insistence of the company itself. Although most companies told us they would rather work with a provider over a period of time to help the provider improve low scores, over half of the large employers we surveyed said if customer service issues continued to be a problem, the providers would be dropped.

"We tend not to be a company that quickly fires our vendors, whether that's in purchasing underwear or purchasing healthcare. We like to work with our vendors, sit down, tell them how we feel, what the problems are, and give them an opportunity to respond. But I think if it [poor scores] went on for a period of time that was unacceptable, then we'd probably fire them," McLeod of J. C. Penney's says.

Although it has not happened yet, Johnson Wax told us that providers who consistently score low in patient satisfaction would not have their contracts renewed.

Giving low-scoring providers the opportunity to improve is important to other companies too. "I can't envision us just saying, 'Gee, here are the criteria and if you don't make it this year, even though you've been with us 15 years, you're out in the cold.' That's not traditionally how we do things," says Robert Wittcoff, director of employee benefits at McDonald's Corporation. "When we develop a partnership, not necessarily only within healthcare, if something goes wrong with that, before we drop vendors we want to help them improve. If the improvement doesn't come, then we'll drop them."

Robert Bonin of First Chicago stresses that dropping a provider, for whatever reason, is not a decision to be entered into lightly, and certainly not without the cooperation of the managed care company itself.

We've taken a role in individual cases where a number of problems have come to our attention. We have done it in the HMO world and have caused people to be decredentialed. The one case I'm thinking of, the HMO wanted to do it anyway. It was a total joining of minds here. We don't know what the doctor was practicing, but it wasn't medicine. Even though he was a big provider for us, he was becoming too expensive. Patients loved him because basically he'd say, "Stay home and complete bed rest for a month or so." Normally we would not get involved at the physician level; we would if it were an exceptional case.

In other instances, employers don't yet have the right or the responsibility to hire or fire a healthcare provider in the system, although that doesn't preclude the company from staying actively involved in the relationship between employee/patient and healthcare provider. At GE, the health plan administrators are required by contract to deal with this issue. "But we expect them to take swift and immediate action." says Bill Ruoff. "From a liability standpoint, we can't add or delete providers." However, he does add that, "If it's a serious complaint, we'll be on the phone with the administrator wanting to know what's happening and explaining that we want an answer on this pretty darn fast. We do give it a sense of immediacy and urgency, but do we control the ultimate decision? No."

THE OTHER SIDE OF THE COIN: COMPANIES DISINTERESTED IN EMPLOYEES' SATISFACTION WITH HEALTHCARE

Although our research shows a clear trend toward greater employer involvement with healthcare customer satisfaction, not every company we interviewed sees the urgent need to get involved. Hallmark Cards, headquartered in Kansas City, Missouri, doesn't survey its employees about healthcare. "We don't do it now and don't plan to do it in the future. Our medical plan means employees have total choice of providers," says Connie Zimmer, insurance benefits manager. Hallmark employees don't report back to the company with their good or their bad healthcare experiences, and if employees become unhappy with the care they receive they simply switch providers themselves.

Another company that doesn't track employee satisfaction with healthcare is Borden, Inc., headquartered in New York City. Borden doesn't survey its employees on healthcare, and has no plans to start doing it in the future, according to Victoria Fortman, director of medical benefits. The company also has no way to track which providers are unpopular among employees. "We would expect the profit centers to let us know, and we would exclude them from future efforts," she says.

The Sara Lee Company in Chicago is another employer that doesn't track employee satisfaction with healthcare. The company may, however, begin tracking that information in the future, according to Jim Clousing, director of employee benefits. He realizes the responsibility employers have to make sure their employees are happy with the care they receive.

And what does he anticipate doing when providers score poorly? "I imagine we'll have to deal with it. I guess we'd have to find out why the remarks are low," he says. For now, a third party deals with it; for example, Aetna Insurance investigates complaints against their providers. "Our employees haven't made many complaints," Clousing says. "In the HMOs and PPOs, they have the choice to go to another doctor."

EMPLOYER INVOLVEMENT IN HEALTHCARE: FUTURE TRENDS

According to Melissa Kennedy, quality issues will become increasingly important as employers delve deeper into the area of employee satisfaction. "Satisfaction is very important to the industry, it's very important to the hospital administrators, it's very important to the employers and the health plans, but they're also becoming more and more interested in the outcomes of these people, not just satisfaction," she says.

From the employers' perspective, it's more than cost that drives their choice of health plans, according to the study's participants. The quality of care offered was ranked highest in terms of priority by employers, followed by access to physicians and cost, a 1995 study found. The study, initiated by the Chicago Business Group on Health, polled 7,000 workers who receive employer-sponsored health insurance through some sort of managed healthcare plan.

Because how much an employee pays for health insurance is largely controlled by employers, not health plans, employers could use results of the study to set pricing strategies, Mindy Kairey, a consultant with Hewitt Associates, told the *Chicago Tribune*.[5] In other words, employers won't simply be asking, "Did you like your hospital and doctor, did you have to wait too long," etc., but questions like, "Are you as active socially now as before your surgery? Can you engage in your social life as much as you used to?" Employers are realizing that patient satisfaction goes beyond what happens in the clinic, physician's office, or hospital.

"This is something that's very important on the part of health plans and employers," says Melissa Kennedy. "They're saying, OK, I know my patients are satisfied and that's great, but is what you're doing to them really helping their quality of life? You replaced their hip, they're satisfied with the hip replacement, but can they walk up and down the steps easier now? And there are tools that allow people to make that assessment," she adds. According to Kennedy, as employers become more involved in employee healthcare, they will eventually do away with the middleman of the

---

5. *Chicago Tribune,* July 5, 1995.

managed care company altogether. For now, employers are most concerned with which plans employees like best. That will change as the employers begin to survey more specific providers. "The employers are not necessarily yet responsible for that [questions about specific doctors]. They just want to find out what health plans are making their employees more satisfied. I don't know that employers are going to be interested in specifically what hospital or doctor until employers have direct relationships with providers, which will happen sooner rather than later, and in effect eliminate the whole health plan/insurance company side of the coin," Kennedy says.

This shift will be the result of integrated health systems, Kennedy says, a concept that has already taken hold at several major corporations. "We've already got very large employers—for example, GTE—who own their own clinics and things, who don't go through insurance companies at all, and they're saving a whole lot of money doing it," she says.

Employers have made quality their next target to improve in healthcare. The momentum has begun to build over the past year and if healthcare costs per employee continue to be as low as they were in 1994 and 1995, employers will focus even more on quality issues. Customer service and patient satisfaction with their providers, based on feedback from their employees, have become their new focus.

3

CHAPTER

Managed Care's Monetary Measures

No aspect of the healthcare revolution has affected more lives, more dramatically, than the introduction of the managed care approach to medical treatment. Since 1985, the number of people enrolled in health maintenance organizations (HMOs) and preferred provider organizations (PPOs) has more than tripled. About 33 percent of the population is covered by an HMO or PPO according to industry research.[1]

A managed care "takeover" of healthcare in the United States will occur between the years 1996 and 2000. Already, about 100 million Americans are enrolled in an HMO or PPO. By the beginning of 1995, every state except Alaska and Wyoming had medical offices of at least one HMO. That marks a dramatic transformation to managed care. For instance, two out of three insured Americans who work in

---

1. SMG Marketing Group, *SMG Market Letter,* August 1993, p. 4; *Estimates for Year 2000* by The Health Forecasting Group.

larger organizations now are enrolled in HMOs and managed care plans, according to a study by KPMG Peat
Marwick of companies with more than 200 employees. For-
profit HMOs grew so rapidly in 1993 and 1994 that they
now enroll more members than do nonprofit plans; and
three-fourths of all physicians have contracts with HMOs
and managed care plans, and 89 percent of physicians
employed in group practices are working under managed
care agreements.[2]

Government health programs will be rapidly converted
into HMOs within the next five years. Medicare and Medicaid will be market targets for HMO enrollment. An estimated 7 percent—or 2.2 million—of the approximately 33
million people eligible for Medicare will have signed up
with HMOs by the end of 1995.[3] As employers push employees into more tightly managed programs and offer increasingly limited choices for healthcare, the issue of ensuring
patient satisfaction has become tantamount to good business. Employers, in exchange for providing such limited
choices, realize they must be able to offer documented proof
to their workers that the benefit plans they are offering to
them will make the employees and their families happy.
That proof comes in the form of customer satisfaction survey results, designed to illustrate what is/is not working
among healthcare providers. Not so long ago, patients followed their physicians to hospitals. But today, pressure to
change hospitals is coming from employees enrolled in
particular health plans.

More frequently health plans are finding that employers listen to their employees as managers choose providers.
Managed care organizations are paying increased attention

2. Eric Eckholm, "While Congress Remains Silent, Healthcare Transforms
   Itself," *The New York Times,* December 18, 1994, pp. A1, 22.
3. SMG Marketing Group, *SMG Market Letter,* August 1993, p. 4; *Estimates
   for Year 2000* by The Health Forecasting Group.

to subscribers' satisfaction with the providers they've chosen. If subscribers aren't happy, they'll likely jump ship to another plan, says Stephen Pew, Ph.D., senior director of improvement information at VHA Inc., Irving, Texas.[4]

During our 1995 research, we spoke with numerous large and midsized managed care organizations that represent more than 25 million employees to determine their approach to tracking and evaluating customer service by their plan providers. The managed care companies themselves are feeling the heat from two sides: the employers, who are demanding good customer service for their employees; and from the patients themselves, who are bonded together in greater numbers, to ensure that their voices are heard. Their message is: *We demand better customer service from our healthcare providers.* One patient told us, "We are getting sick and tired of being ill treated!"

COMPETITION'S FOCUS ON CUSTOMER SERVICE

The directors of managed care companies have seen this trend developing and are realizing how important customer service is, and will continue to be. "That's going to be one of the number one things—trying to maintain your patient base," acknowledges Nan Wallis, executive director of American Lifecare in New Orleans, a PPO with an enrollment of 340,000. "With as many health plans as there are out there, everyone's going to have to improve on customer satisfaction, service, and everything else."

The principle reason for this new focus, quite simply, is price. "I think the price of healthcare, proportionately, will continue to fall. In other words, as everyone is tightening their belt and delivery of medical care becomes locked into cap rates, and premium prices don't continue to rise

---

4. *Hospitals & Health Network,* December 5, 1994, p. 68.

the way they were, I think you're going to see people fighting to stay in line, pricing-wise, to stay competitive. The differentiating factor is going to be customer and client service," says Wallis.

Paul Gardetto agrees. "The way we've decided to differentiate ourselves within this market is through service, because somebody else is setting the prices. So we take this stuff very seriously," says Gardetto, service assurance manager at Humana Wisconsin Health Organization in Milwaukee, Wisconsin, an HMO with 100,000 subscribers. "Customer-satisfaction scores will be a very important piece of the decision making process," says David Epstein, MD, Prudential's vice president of medical services for its southern group in Atlanta.

Dr. Epstein says customer satisfaction will become even more important in managed-care selection when hospitals competing for contracts standardize their measuring tools. Currently, HMOs find it difficult to compare hospital scores because different survey techniques are used, he says.[5]

Everyone in the managed care arena seems to agree that change is in the air. But not everyone in the medical community is so quick to embrace this brave new world. "It's very difficult because if there is a profession that's couched in tradition and won't budge, it's medicine," says Robert Herek, director of customer service for Cigna Healthcare of Arizona, an HMO with half a million members, located in Phoenix. "Really, it's embarrassing sometimes how we are set in our ways. When we look at ourselves we don't think so, but when others look at us, it's big-time."

The healthcare revolution of the past decade has affected each component of the healthcare equation: consumer, provider, and payer. One major result of this change has been the increased interaction of the employer with the health plan itself, which may be a factor of increased customer awareness, according to Tom Beggs, senior research

---

5. *Modern Healthcare*, July 18, 1994, p. 30.

associate for IHC-Inter-Mountain Health Care, an HMO/
PPO of half a million members in the Salt Lake City area.

> I think that with the competitiveness of the industry,
> consumers are awakening to the fact that they need to
> be more involved in the consumption of this product.
> Average Americans know more about their toaster than
> they do about their healthcare plan. And that's coming
> to the front, and the big companies are saying, "Gee, we
> can't afford to continue to keep paying X number of
> dollars in premiums a year. What can we all do together
> to help contain the costs?" Part of that is the insured
> waking up and saying, "Well, I really don't need to see
> a specialist for this. I'm going to go to my GP first and
> see if this ear infection is anything other than swimmer's
> ear." Rather than running off to an ENT at three or four
> or five hundred dollars a pop; or worse yet, going to the
> emergency room on the weekend to do it because you
> don't want to wait until Monday morning.

This increased consumer awareness goes hand in hand
with increased pressure from the employer, who is asking
for information about specific providers within the health
plan network. Says Beggs:

> Client companies are saying to us, "What information do
> you have about this plan, that plan, and the providers
> in those plans?" We are saying internally, "Hmm, I
> wonder, why does one physician have a full service, the
> other doesn't?" One sees X number of patients a day, the
> other sees $2X$ patients a day, and so forth. So we're just
> sort of digging around, looking at that information. It's
> information that we need in order to be more efficient in
> management.

HOW MANAGED CARE COMPANIES MEASURE PATIENT SATISFACTION

A full 100 percent of the managed care companies we interviewed in the summer of 1995 either survey their members or plan to do so in the future. The methods they use

to measure patient satisfaction vary. For instance, 76 percent of those interviewed use mail-in surveys, 65 percent
do phone surveys, 6 percent use a file of complaints, and
6 percent use focus groups.

Many managed care companies realize that the issue
of customer satisfaction within a health plan can be broken
down into two components: clinical quality and service
quality. Says Gardetto of Humana:

> To satisfy the member, which is the customer, both the
> provider customer and the member customer, there are
> really two ways that they measure quality. One is, "Is
> the doctor nice? Does the receptionist treat me well? Did
> I get seen in a reasonable amount of time, and was the
> care appropriate?" That kind of thing. But it's also, "Do
> my claims get paid on time?" "Do I get put on hold when
> I call Humana?" So it's, "How am I treated as a cus-
> tomer?" So we split it into service quality issues and
> clinical quality issues.

Many managed care companies make this distinction
in tracking and analyzing their survey results. Traditionally, surveys focused more on the service quality side of
satisfaction, but more managed care companies today realize that the two issues go hand-in-hand: Good service
quality impacts good clinical quality, and vice versa.

Many of the managed care companies we interviewed
have only recently begun to track patient satisfaction information down to the level of satisfaction with individual
providers. But to many people in the industry, it makes
sense for managed care companies to elicit the most specific
information possible when the companies survey their
members about satisfaction. "Think about the stakeholders
and their different perceptions," offers Melissa Kennedy,
vice president of HealthCare Research Systems at Ohio
State University. "The health plans want to know who the
providers of care are that make people happy, because they

want those providers on their panel, and they want providers who don't make patients satisfied off their panel, so I think insurance companies are asking more and more those types of questions," Kennedy says.

Because the customer service revolution in healthcare is just warming up, it does mean that long-term statistics about patient satisfaction trends are nonexistent. For many managed care companies, this translates into some uncertainty about which programs are the most, or least, successful. "You don't really know until you can look back on 5 or 10 years and say, 'Yeah, that helped here,' or, 'We need to do more of this there,' or whatever it happens to be," says Tom Beggs. "But you have to try. You can't just sit back and say, 'Gee, I hope we're doing the right thing.' "

Some industry experts feel the managed care industry manipulates the data from enrollees to make themselves look better and misses the valuable points altogether. Roberta Clarke, an associate professor of healthcare management at Boston university, says managed-care organizations are losing enrollees at a rate of about 20 percent a year, a rate she says would be "truly horrendous" in other industries. Moreover, she states HMOs, PPOs, and point-of-service plans aren't tracking data that could help stop the dramatic customer loss.

Clarke called about 25 managed care organizations for an ongoing study, but most lacked precise disenrollment figures, including voluntary versus involuntary disenrollment.

She also accuses managed care organizations of "playing footsie" with customer-satisfaction data. "In every ad I've ever seen for a managed-care organization, the customer-satisfaction rate is always in the high 90s", she says. "It makes you wonder: Where are all those managed care organizations that people are complaining about?" She urges managed care organizations to empower their marketers to study and track disenrollment and customer satisfaction and to focus on access, coverage and customer service rather than promotion.[6]

MANAGED CARE'S USE OF PATIENT FEEDBACK TO IMPROVE CUSTOMER SERVICE

The results of patient satisfaction surveys are often used to counsel hospitals and individual physicians, and a growing percentage of the managed care companies we spoke to use satisfaction scores as part of a physician's contract negotiation or as part of a bonus package. For example, in FHP of Colorado, top-performing providers receive an incentive of 40 cents per member per month, according to Lori Muneta, research analyst. In 50 percent of the companies interviewed, a provider may be dropped from the network for continued poor scores.

In other cases, managed care companies use their survey results as the impetus to help devise new and better programs for customer service. For example, Humana has recently begun a new initiative for hiring customer service representatives called Care Coordinators. In this new program, every person who answers the telephone at Humana will be a care coordinator, and every one of them will be a college graduate who will be considered part of the management team. "In the past, usually the person answering the phone was the lowest-paid person on the totem pole," explains Paul Gardetto. "That just doesn't make sense. Now they'll be some of the highest-paid people. Because that's how we interface with our customer. It's going to be expensive, but hopefully it will pay off."

In other cases, managed care companies use their survey results to solve problems that they might never have known about if it hadn't been brought to their attention through a survey. For example, the Provider Relations

---

6. *Modern Healthcare*, July 17, 1995.

Department at Health Service Network in Cincinnati, Ohio, recently came across a survey filled out by a young man whose wife had died during childbirth. "When he filled out the survey, he indicated that he had no clue what had happened medically," explains Barbara Kauffman, director of marketing for the 1.5 million-member PPO. "Now, we're not sure if the doctors and the staff failed to share that information with him or if he was too distraught to understand it. He never received his wife's autopsy report. Our advocate worked with him to direct him back to the physician to get some of those answers, and to work with the physicians to facilitate that response. The issue was ultimately resolved," she says.

Some managed care organizations will use their data to impact provider compensation and or bonus programs. A study of 200 HMO medical directors was conducted in 1995, by National Research Corp., a Lincoln, Nebraska-based market research firm. Of the HMOs collecting physician data, 60 percent are using the scores as part of a physician compensation/bonus program. Extrapolated over the entire sample of HMOs, 36 percent are assessing patient satisfaction with individual physicians and using the findings to help determine physician pay.

The larger the HMO, the more likely the data will be used as part of a compensation/bonus program. Some 70 percent of HMOs with 50,000 or more enrollees use the information for compensation programs. At HMOs with fewer than 50,000 enrollees, it drops to 50 percent.

THE MANAGED CARE PERSPECTIVE: WHAT DO PATIENTS WANT?

As our research demonstrated in Chapter 1, when it comes to good patient relations and customer service, the simplest issues are by far the most important. A caring, compassionate hospital staff and physician will always rank highly in patient satisfaction surveys. This simple truth is realized by the people at the Cigna Healthcare headquarters in Bloomfield, Connecticut. "The satisfaction levels are highest with those providers who take the time to treat patients like individuals, not treat them like just one more file," says Sali Bonazelli, director of Cigna Healthcare Marketing.

That personal touch is important to patients, managed care companies realize. But along with that comes a growing realization that the customer comes first; that the doctor works for the patient, and not vice versa. Says Herek of Cigna in Phoenix:

> I think a lot of us give lip service to the statement, "We must know the needs of our customers, and provide service either at those expectation levels or greater than that." But look at something as basic as operating hours. If you go back to when those hours were originally set as being from eight to five, those hours were set for the convenience of the physician, way back when. And now we, the customer, believe that those are the hours we set, and we believe that we are asking for favors if we say, "Couldn't you keep your clinics open later than five o'clock?"

To Herek, those old standards no longer make sense in today's two-career, nontraditional family world. "When you look at the economy and the two bread-winner families, with both spouses working to put weenies and beans on the table, we realize we better start paying attention to customer service. And if we're going to ask the questions, we better be prepared for the answers," he says.

Survey results have shown that a big concern for members in an HMO or PPO is the fear of not having the opportunity to choose your own doctor. But that isn't as much of a problem as many people may think, according to Tom Beggs of IHC in Salt Lake City.

> There are a lot of misperceptions out there. There's a general perception, even in our company, that people are less satisfied with the more tightly managed program

with an HMO. That in fact is opposite. Both in national surveys and in the surveys we do here, we find out that people are much more satisfied who are on HMO plans than people who are on PPOs or indemnity plans. After you drag them into the HMO kicking and screaming, complaining that there's only 600 physicians to choose from on the panel, they get in there and 99 percent end up with a doctor that they like. Some of course just never will, and they'll keep hopping around from doctor to doctor. But they get in there, they get to know that person, and they get to like him or her. As long as we don't take off the wrong leg, like they did in Florida, we've got smooth sailing. They [members] know that whenever they go, it's going to be a ten-dollar copay or a five-dollar copay, or in some cases, no copay, and that's that. And these plans all have out-of-pocket caps, usually $1,000 per person, $2,000 per family. So you know that in a worst-case scenario, you're going to have to come up with $2,000 over the course of a year. We rarely ever have to deal with that. And if your doctor isn't there, there are emergency considerations, urgent care considerations. It's one-stop shopping. And it works.

THE PROBLEM OF LOW-SCORING PROVIDERS: WHAT WILL MANAGED CARE COMPANIES DO?

Although many managed care companies are willing to take drastic action with low-scoring providers—even terminating them when necessary—most stress the educational aspect of working with providers, and giving them every possible opportunity to improve their performance before such radical actions are undertaken.

Nearly half of the managed care organizations we interviewed stated that they would drop providers who flunk the customer service standards they set. Two of the largest, Kaiser Permanente and Humana, said they would drop providers if necessary. Kaiser, which serves 6.6 million enrollees in 16 states and the District of Columbia, indicated

that in some markets, a consistently low-scoring provider
is dropped from the group. Humana, with 3.3 million
enrollees, said the organization will try to find out what's
wrong, educate the provider, but drop him or her if the need
dictates.

Prudential currently is less likely to change providers,
but that may change. "Right now, we wouldn't change a
provider unless there were serious questions about customer service," Dr. Epstein says. "But with newly created
networks or realigned networks, customer satisfaction could
be an important piece of information that differentiates one
hospital from another."[7]

"When we attack an issue, we don't attack the 'who,'
we attack the 'what,' " says Gardetto of Humana. "Providers
want to do a good job. Ninety-nine percent of them don't
have an agenda other than treating their patient." However, problems do sometimes occur. "If the providers are
subaverage performers, we either need to educate them or
get rid of them. And we'll do any one of those actions. We
do put pressure on the providers for price, and for what we
expect of them. So they obviously have got something in-
vested in this, too," Gardetto states.

At Preferred Health Care Inc., in Wichita, Kansas,
low-scoring providers receive two warnings before being
dropped from the network. But providers have a strong
incentive not to let that happen, and once again that incentive comes down to dollars and cents. "Once they get one
or two warnings, they don't want out of our network because we're the largest network in the Wichita area. They
can't afford to lose our business," says Gaylee Dolloff, vice
president of program services at Preferred Health Care, an
HMO with an enrollment of 108,000 and a network of 900
physicians.

Beech Street of California, which tracks customer service issues like "friendliness and cheerfulness" of providers

7. *Modern Healthcare*, July 18, 1994, p. 30.

staff, told us that if low marks continue with a provider they will be dropped from the program. Bob Gerger, controller for the PPO, which has 8.8 million enrollees said, "Negative responses weigh a great deal. If that [negative feedback from the patient] continues, then it becomes an issue with us as to whether we want to keep that provider in the network." The Prudential said they will terminate providers who do not improve, whereas FHP of Colorado will deny bonus fees to low scorers.

Although tracking patient satisfaction is something most managed care organizations have been doing for years, the major difference now is they are going to do something more drastic with the data. More and more, as pressure mounts from the employers, they will use the customer service information to choose providers, in contract negotiations, and to help determine provider bonuses. Customer service performance by providers will undoubtedly be tied to monetary rewards more and more as the patient satisfaction revolution gains momentum.

4
CHAPTER

Competing Means
Satisfying Patients

"A poorly designed patient satisfaction survey can be worse
than not measuring patient satisfaction at all, it can actually be harmful to a provider, particularly if it gives them
false-positive results. They'll swear they're doing well until
the day they are forced to close their doors due to unresolved patient satisfaction issues." Irwin Press, PhD and cofounder of Press-Ganey, Inc., doesn't mince words, and he
believes that developing a patient satisfaction survey is
both art and science.

"Slowly the industry is realizing it has to compete, and
successfully competing in healthcare means satisfying
patients," says Dr. Press. His firm helped Mercy Hospital
Medical Center in Des Moines, Iowa, identify problems in
its emergency department (ED) and has worked actively in
the healthcare industry measuring patient satisfaction since
1985. Press-Ganey, Inc., currently serves more than 500
clients. "If you satisfy patients, they're less likely to sue you,
they're more likely to come back, and they're more likely
to recommend you to others." Press believes that it's essential

that hospitals find out where they can improve, and then take action. "Survey data is meaningless unless you use it and when you use it, you can make a difference."

Management at Mercy Hospital Medical Center understood that people don't usually go to hospital emergency rooms by choice; what they didn't understand was that extended wait times made patients feel as though they were "being ignored." Most of us know the feeling. It's frustrating, but getting angry just doesn't seem like the appropriate response. And for some reason, you start to notice negative details you might otherwise overlook.

That was exactly what was happening at Mercy. In January 1992, managers reviewing patient survey data noted that long waits and limited medical staff scrambling to care for the sickest patients were taking their toll on Mercy's patient satisfaction ratings. There was no significant increase in complaints, just increasingly frustrated patients. The patterns were clear, and after reviewing alternatives, hospital managers concluded it was time to make a change. As a result, the hospital opened a minor care unit to treat patients with less serious conditions and regrouped nurses into teams to make them accountable for certain patients. Those actions raised scores on subsequent surveys and boosted staff morale. "Obviously, satisfaction and quality are in the eyes of the user," says Pat Spurlock, administrative director of the emergency department. "Until you listen to your patients, you're not going to know whether you're meeting their needs."

Patient satisfaction surveys like the one for Mercy summarized in Table 4.1 not only help target improvements in services but can become a part of continuous quality improvement efforts. But now, increasing managed care penetration is changing old assumptions about patient choice of hospitals and underscoring the importance of the patient satisfaction survey as an important tool.[1]

---

1. "Are Patients Happy? Managed Care Plans Want to Know," *Hospitals & Health Networks,* December 5, 1994, p. 68.

TABLE 4.1

Selected Results from Mercy Hospital Medical Center's Patient
Satisfaction Surveys

	Satisfaction Rates	
Factor Surveyed	**January 1992** **(%)**	**July 1994** **(%)**
1. Courtesy of the hospital's nurses	79	88
2. Technical skill of the nurses	84	86

Source: "Are Patients Happy? Managed Care Plans Want to Know," *Hospitals & Health Networks*,
December 5, 1994, p. 68.

MANAGED CARE FIRMS LISTEN TO PATIENTS

"Not so long ago, patients followed their physicians to
hospitals. But today, pressure to change hospitals is coming
from employees enrolled in particular health plans. Managed care organizations are paying increased attention to
subscribers' satisfaction with the providers they've chosen.
If subscribers aren't happy, they'll likely jump ship to
another plan," says Stephen Pew, PhD, senior director of
improvement information at VHA Inc., in Irving, Texas.

According to Melissa Kennedy at HealthCare Research
Systems, a patient satisfaction survey company affiliated
with Ohio State University, "Employers and health plans
are dying for this data because they're using it at the
negotiation table."

Patient satisfaction surveys not only help target improvements in services but can become a part of continuous
quality improvement efforts. The Joint Commission on
Accreditation of Healthcare Organizations (JCAHO) has
incorporated requirements to measure patient satisfaction
and "meet its expectations" within their 1995 standards. As
a result, there is a lot of activity in the patient satisfaction
survey business. Some hospital patient surveys are done in-
house; others are conducted by outside firms. The VHA,

with its 1,000 affiliates, is developing a patient satisfaction survey for its hospitals. The alliance is exploring a variety of survey methods: telephone calls, mailback forms, and computerized systems. The Agency for Health Care Policy and Research recently hired a research institute to develop a model instrument for a consumer survey. The goal was to develop a consensus on which kinds of consumer satisfaction and consumer perception information should be collected and surveyed. The research involves exploring questions that look at hospitals and how hospitals choices interact with a choice of health plans.

We looked closely at three firms, all using different formats, client bases, and research approaches to get a better idea of a provider's alternatives:

> Press-Ganey, considered one of the pioneers in the industry, with more than 500 participating clients, recommends that surveys be mailed to patients within a few days of discharge. Their base survey contains 49 questions, but hospitals can customize the survey to meet their specific needs. The surveys are designed for different specialties, such as day surgery, emergency departments, ambulatory care, and home care.

> HealthCare Research Systems, a group of professionals affiliated with Ohio State University, believes the firm has two sets of clients: employers and providers. Although the firm conducts conventional surveys, similar in format to those employed by Press-Ganey, it also performs "quick assessments" for employers (like Xerox, Digital, GTE, and GE) and health plans (recently the firm completed a survey of more than 30,000 patients for Kaiser-Permanente). They use mailback, telephone, and computer-based survey formats.

> The Picker Institute, a nonprofit affiliate of the Beth Israel Corporation, adopted a mission to promote

healthcare quality assessment and improvement strategies that address patients' needs and concerns as defined by patients. The institute has surveyed more than 45,000 patients and their families, and has worked with more than 200 healthcare institutions and community healthcare coalitions. In addition to global ratings using a four or five point scale, Picker/Commonwealth surveys also ask patients to report whether specific events took place. The institute staff believe these simple reporting variations provide managers with the ability to identify problems without having to analyze time variations in ratings.

Finally, we reviewed dozens of surveys designed internally by healthcare institutions. Although formats were sometimes similar, each seemed to have unique characteristics that reflected the particular focus of the institution involved. Their uniqueness may have been both their greatest strength and most significant weakness. Although they provided specific data—excellent for providing a time series comparison—it was not possible to compare the data to other institutions of similar size, patient base, or regional dispersion.

Survey Format

Clearly, all surveys prepared by the three companies we reviewed recognized the need to specialize survey questions based on the services used:

- *Inpatient surveys* designed for the areas of medicine, surgery, childbirth, and pediatrics.
- *Ambulatory/outpatient surveys* designed for all aspects of ambulatory care.
- *Emergency services surveys* that identify the unique aspects of urgent care.

- *Homecare surveys* detailing issues like care instruction and coordination of services.

Press-Ganey has developed a coordinated and complete set of instruments, whereas the Picker Institute is still in the development stage for all but the inpatient and ambulatory survey products.

HealthCare Research Associates will design an instrument based on the specific needs of the client, and many times the client is not the hospital. When the consultants work with employers, they start by asking questions about the overall benefits package, then move to the specifics of their patient care. Beyond specifics of delivery of care, consultants also focus on these three areas:

- Do employees have access to the doctors they want?
- Can they get an appointment at their PCP (primary care provider) when needed?
- Do they feel that the dollars paid for coverage is appropriate?

All these things create the employee's or member's perception of satisfaction with the health plan *before* they even see a doctor!

All Questions Are *Not* the Same

Stephen Strasser, PhD and executive director of HealthCare Research Systems, feels it is essential that survey questions be absolutely balanced. Here is a sample question from an HCRS survey:

Parking was not a problem. a. *Strongly Disagree*
b. *Disagree*
c. *Neither Agree*
   nor Disagree
d. *Agree*
e. *Strongly Agree*

Strasser points out that each response has a balanced "contraresponse"— "Strongly disagree" is the exact opposite of "strongly agree." "Disagree" is the opposite of "agree." "Neither agree nor disagree" is a neutral response.

Strasser adds, "We would not use a term like 'excellent,' because it can produce a false positive response. There is not an obvious 'contraresponse' to 'excellent' and as a result, questions are often structured with more positive responses than potentially negative responses." For example, the following question was taken from a survey developed in a 400-bed facility in Pontiac, Michigan:

> *The compassion shown by the staff was*   *a. Excellent*
> *b. Very Good*
> *c. Good*
> *d. Fair*
> *e. Poor*

Of the five available responses, four are generally favorable. Strasser's perspective is that a question like this is much more likely to produce a positive patient response than a balanced response. He points out that although that may be good for an administrator's ego, it does little to identify real patient satisfaction issues within the organization.

Survey Methods: Timing Is Everything

After exploring a variety of survey methods, the 1,000-member VHA hospital alliance believes that the optimal moment to survey patients is 14 to 30 days after discharge. The VHA asserts that it is still recent enough for the patient to recall most aspects of his/her experience but long enough to provide perspective to the incident requiring healthcare services. Press-Ganey recommends that its clients mail surveys one to three days after discharge. HealthCare Research Systems is less specific but has actually developed "point-of-service" computer survey systems that enable

patients to comment on service levels almost as the services
are provided.

Patient satisfaction survey data is collected by consulting firms through three primary methods:

- Mailback surveys.
- Telephone interviews.
- On-site surveys and computer systems.

Given the same questionnaire, former patients will go
easier on the provider if their comments are taken over the
phone or face to face, rather than on a mailed survey. The
scores for telephone surveys not only fail to capture the
extreme dissatisfaction that may be out there but may also
yield a narrower spread of opinion than with a written
survey that's mailed back.

The choice of data collection method can mean a de-
ceptively rosier and less detailed picture for healthcare
providers, which can complicate efforts to fix problems before
they result in customer defections. Melvin Hall, PhD, author of the study that disclosed these findings, cautions
providers not to be lulled into false confidence. To be effective, a survey must be able to ensure two things: that the
sample is representative of the population being targeted
and that the survey procedure encourages open and honest
evaluations.

Those who promote the phone method say it usually
yields a much higher response rate, which reduces the
likelihood that the results are unrepresentative of the target
population. However, phone surveys contain an "acquies-
cence bias" or a tendency to agree with what's being asked
by a phone interviewer. "Patients are intimidated by
healthcare and caregivers," according to Hall. "They are
less inclined to criticize the hospital when contacted in
person." Mailed responses showed a wider range of responses—more results at the lower end of the scale but also
a good representation of former patients who were extremely
satisfied. The diverse scores reflect a greater degree of

thought that leads to more elaborate and useful feedback. In addition, "The mailback method seems more likely to garner opinions of those most critical of the care received." The value to the institution is that administrators have a better chance to hear those who have reservations about their care, giving them an opportunity to improve.

Trending Reports, Summary Reports, and Reports on Reports

All survey companies provide for extensive and comprehensive summary reports. However, volume and value are not synonymous. The Picker Institute stresses the "actionable" nature of their reports. While most patient satisfaction instruments are designed to generate global impressions of various aspects of care, Picker/Commonwealth survey questions are designed to generate information that managers can act upon. Their questions differ from the other two survey companies in that in addition to perception ratings, they detail whether specific events took place (that is, information provided about medication side effects, follow-up visits, or delays in scheduling). This type of response reporting can sometimes make it easier for managers to identify problems without having to analyze variations in ratings.

Press-Ganey's extensive client base offers the most flexible peer groupings, providing meaningful normative comparisons. Perhaps the most useful tool in its quarterly report package is an executive summary that identifies major changes (both positive and negative) from previous periods. Clients are able to quickly focus on potential problem areas.

HealthCare Research Systems has a unique reporting/database analysis tool that enables clients to "interact" with patient responses. HCRS has the ability to correlate patient medical records with patient satisfaction responses. As a result, it is feasible to identify which floors, physicians, nursing stations, and procedures (as well as virtually unlimited analysis groupings) produce the most positive and negative results.

ARE WE MEASURING THE RIGHT THINGS?

Clearly, providers, employers, and health plans have access to sophisticated patient satisfaction instruments that are statistically valid and useful in determining whether healthcare institutions are providing a reasonably high quality of services. However, the instruments consistently measured only the level of satisfaction associated with the current provider's procedures and services. In other words, it is generally communicated to the patient that "these are the things we do (or are supposed to do); please tell us how you think we did those things." Therefore, this approach is likely to produce the same potentially "false positives" we are attempting to avoid by carefully structuring our questions.

The next step may be to "break out of the box" and ask patients what they expected, or perhaps more importantly, what they wanted. Then, based on their response, we can ask how close we came.

Only then can providers truly determine whether they are meeting their patients' needs.

5

CHAPTER

Angry Patients Want Dramatic Improvements

Because almost every person surveyed in our 1995 study said that customer service by their hospital and physician was "extremely important," we asked patients to define customer service in a healthcare setting. We got a passionate response, with answers ranging from the emotional to the profound:

- "They should treat you like a human being—like you matter."
- "Just listen to the patients. Listen to what they say, as well as what they don't say."
- "Have empathy for my feelings, my confusion, my fears, my pain."

But we also heard another message. Many told us loudly and clearly that they are angry. Patients said they are sick and tired of being treated like they are an intrusion in a healthcare worker's day. A pet peeve is endless wait time spent in emergency rooms, registration areas, radiology departments, and doctors' offices. And while patients wait, they are observing what they believe to be inefficiencies and inappropriate employee activities.

We interviewed and surveyed nearly 2,000 people in 17 states who had received care from 30 hospitals and hundreds of physician offices within the last year. We asked how important customer service was to them. Not surprisingly, 90 percent of those who responded said it was "extremely important" in physicians' offices. We also asked them to define customer service in their own words, as well as rate their recent experiences with all types of healthcare providers. When we asked patients to rate their most recent hospital stay, the average score was 7.4 on a 10-point scale. On its surface, this is a respectable, "average" rating, until you look a little closer. Unfortunately for hospitals and clinics, many patients don't grade customer service on a "curve."

Nearly a third of the patients gave their hospitals a "failing grade" of less than 5 on that 10-point index. Patients are not expecting perfection. When asked what the rating should have been, the same patients replied that the score should have been as high as 9.4 on a 10-point scale. Sometimes it was simply a matter of courtesy that patients found lacking in a hospital staff. "Every morning they would get me up at 5 AM to weigh me. I could always hear them coming down the hallway, even though they tried to be quiet. But to this day, I can't understand why it was necessary to wake me up at that hour, just to weigh me. I don't think I got a good night's sleep the entire time I was in the hospital."

And at other times, the lack of communication created more serious concerns: "I was asked to sign a consent form without a clear explanation of what I was authorizing. In my opinion, 'informed consent' means exactly what it says. I was not informed and did not understand the biopsy procedure that was subsequently performed. I was upset and angry."

A less frequent complaint, but one cited sufficiently to evidence concern by patients, is related to the technical competence of the staff: "I repeatedly observed inappropriate actions by one of the nurses: one person, not the entire staff. However, both my wife and I observed the same person. I asked that he not come to my room. Unfortunately, he was sent anyway."

Although clinics and physician offices fared slightly better, they still only averaged an 8.2 rating, with more than a quarter of their patients rating them at 5 or less. The clear frustration in physicians' offices is excessive wait time: "Had to wait two hours to be seen at a local clinic. When I complained, I was told they had misplaced my records and were 'working on it.'" Sometimes the wait time can be more than frustrating; at times it can impact the level of care provided to the patient: "I will never forget waiting in the OB/gyne examination room, stripped down— cold and frightened—for more than an hour. Finally, I simply got dressed and left. I never even saw a physician."

MANY PATIENTS WILL NOT RETURN TO A HOSPITAL

Hospital patients from across the country indicated that almost 4 out of 10 are unhappy with the billing and collection process. The survey revealed that 6 percent of the patients were so disappointed with billing and collection procedures that they would not return to the same hospital for future care or recommend it to others. This means hospitals are losing more than 6 percent of future revenue for reasons that could be avoided.

From simply understanding hospital charges displayed on the bill to explanation of insurance, more than 35 percent of the patients were dissatisfied. Of these, 10 percent were extremely dissatisfied. Low patient satisfaction levels heavily contribute to a hospital's archnemesis: delayed cash flow and patient complaints.

So, why are so many patients so disenchanted about billing and collection? A common excuse is that healthcare billing is too complex and certainly not user-friendly. Regarding requests for further information about billing questions or problems, about 30 percent of the respondents said they were not happy with the assistance they had received. Patients were not satisfied with the ability of the billing representatives to understand their questions and provide answers or solutions; many former patients complained about the speed with which an answer/solution was given. The unfriendliness of the representative was also a cause for discontent. In analyzing patient responses, poor perception of the billing and collection process was closely related to the lack of up-front information about the reimbursement process. More than one-third of all patients received no information about insurance billing during the registration process, at time of discharge, or during insurance billing.

YOUNGER PATIENTS HAVE THE HIGHEST EXPECTATIONS AND LOWEST PERCEPTION OF SERVICE

As we tried to understand the patient's perspective, we observed another interesting phenomenon. As Table 5.1 shows, older patients (over 55) are less likely to be critical of their healthcare provider than middle-aged patients (36 to 55). Not only did older patients rate hospitals and physicians higher overall, they were significantly less likely to score the provider five or less.

Younger patients (those under 35) have the highest expectations and lowest perception of healthcare delivery. This data, summarized in Table 5.2, suggests that employers and managed care providers have good reason to be concerned about future customer service ratings.

TABLE 5.1

Rating of Customer Service by Age Group

	Older Patients	Middle-Aged Patients
Rating of last hospital experience*	7.9	6.8
Ratings at less than 50%	27%	32%

*Rating scale 1 = low, 10 = high.

TABLE 5.2

Rating of Customer Service by the Under-35 Age Group

	Younger Patients (Under 35)
Rating of last hospital experience:	6.7
Where it should have been:	9.6
Rating of last clinic experience:	7.7
Where it should have been:	9.4

Leading the "customer service revolution in healthcare" are younger and middle-aged patients—those currently in the work force, ultimately paying the bills. They are dissatisfied with current service levels and have their own perception of what is "appropriate" care.

A February 1995 study by *Consumer Reports* pointed to one other dimension of patient satisfaction. That organization's database related the condition being treated to the patient's happiness with care, service, and personnel. Table 5.3 shows the percentage of patients who were dissatisfied with their healthcare provider. Interestingly, the ailments topping the list are not necessarily the most serious, but instead those for which a clear treatment program is often lacking. When questioned, respondents stated

TABLE 5.3

Percentage of Patients Dissatisfied with Provider—by Ailments

Condition Treated	Patient Dissatisfaction (%)
Chronic Headache	23
Lower Back Pain	20
Broken Bones, Torn Ligaments	18
Anxiety, Depression	17
Arthritis	15
Intestinal or Stomach Problems	15
Pregnancy	13
Allergy	12
Respiratory Problems	11
Cancer	11
Prostate Problems (not cancer)	10
Heart Condition	10
Diabetes	8
High Blood Pressure	8
Cataracts or Glaucoma	8
High Cholesterol	7

*Source: "How Is Your Doctor Treating You?" Copyright 1995 by Consumers Union of U.S., Inc., Yonkers, NY 10703-1057. Reprinted by permission from *Consumer Reports*, February 1995, p. 82.

they often felt "left out" of the treatment program. They didn't understand what the physician and/or caregiver was trying to accomplish, and didn't know how to become more involved in their own care.

A clear message of the analysis seems to be the value of ongoing communication between the patient and the caregiver. The importance of communication was confirmed by our own survey results.

SURVEY RESULTS FOR ASPECTS OF CUSTOMER SERVICE

We asked patients to describe "customer service" within a hospital in their own words. We then attempted to classify their responses into major categories shown in Table 5.4.

TABLE 5.4

Patient Definition of Customer Service by Hospitals

What Patients Want	National Average	Older Patients (over 55)	Middle-Aged Patients (36 to 55)	Younger Patients (under 35)
Compassion	40.5%	39.5%	38.7%	40.0%
Communication	40.5	31.6	58.1	26.7
Shorter Wait Time	39.3	50.0	22.6	46.7
Friendliness	36.9	36.9	29.0	53.3
Professionalism	25.0	15.8	22.6	46.7
Efficiency	15.5	21.1	9.7	13.3
Accuracy	7.1	10.5	3.2	6.7
Privacy	4.8	7.9	3.2	3.1

Patients were able to identify more than one area, so totals exceed 100%.

Interestingly, core competencies like efficiency, accuracy, and privacy appear to be expected, and they did not often represent a significant aspect of a patient's customer service perception.

Communication

At or near the top of the list for nearly all age groups were communication and compassion. For some, they were characterized by simple consideration for another person's time: "The hospital took the time to call us and say they were running a little behind, and suggested we come later, so we wouldn't have to wait." For some, the feeling is just as strong, but not nearly as positive: "My wife was treated like a 'customer' instead of a 'patient'—and that's exactly the problem. Hospitals seem to be run by people with business degrees, with an eye on making a profit first instead of combining patient care with cost." And many others acknowledged a special person who was able to communicate a high level of compassion or professionalism: "I had wonderful service, especially from a wonderful, kind RN on the second shift." "Dr. Green performed knee surgery on me. He was so professional but yet made me feel so comfortable. He had excellent bedside manner, second to none." "Had good, qualified nurses in intensive care area, continually watched my progress and made me feel they were really concerned about me."

As indicated in the first portion of the chapter, it is clear that patients from different age groups have different ideas of the most important aspects of customer service. Middle-aged patients mentioned the importance of communication in almost 60 percent of their responses (Table 5.5), significantly higher than any other age group.

A lapse in communication, regardless of how subtle or unintended, can have a disturbing impact on patient care and is likely to remain in the patient's memory for a long time: "There was a miscommunication between me and the doctor regarding the medication used after delivery. I ended up in tremendous pain for three to four hours. He thought he was saving me money; he may have saved money, but I paid for it differently."

One of our respondents pointed out that good communication doesn't always mean telling the patient everything: "I really didn't want to know all the details. I told the doctor I'd ask if I wanted to know; otherwise, he should just tell me what he wanted me to do. We're all different you know. He respected my wishes, and I appreciated that."

Wait Times

We weren't surprised to see that elderly patients were concerned about excessive wait time (Table 5.6): "I was told to come in at 1 PM, to find out that 12 other patients had been told to arrive at the same time."

TABLE 5.5

Percentage of Patients Mentioning Importance of Communication

	Average	**Older**	**Middle**	**Younger**
Communication	40.5%	31.6%	58.1%	26.7%

TABLE 5.6

Percentage of Patients Mentioning Importance of Wait Time

	Average	**Older**	**Middle**	**Younger**
Wait Time	39.3%	50.0%	22.6%	46.7%

(Elderly patients also commented frequently regarding the difficulty associated with accessing a facility's services; parking, valet service, and long hallways without hand rails.)

Perhaps more interesting is how often wait time was cited by younger patients (46.7 percent) as a key aspect of customer satisfaction. "At Children's, even when left in a waiting room for a short time, we were told 'your wait will be. . . .' It was great knowing we hadn't been forgotten."

When wait time was excessive, it often resulted in an unsatisfactory rating of the entire experience: "I was left for hours in a waiting room in ER while doctors and nurses were sitting, doing nothing."

As Table 5.7 shows, wait time becomes one of the most important dimensions of customer service when patients consider their expectations at a clinic or physician's office.

TABLE 5.7

Patients' Definition of Customer Service by Physician

What Patients Want	National Average	Older Patients (over 55)	Middle-Aged Patients (36 to 55)	Younger Patients (under 35)
Shorter Wait Time	52.3%	60.0%	43.3%	46.7%
Friendliness of Staff	41.9	42.5	33.3	60.0
Communication	44.2	37.5	56.7	40.0
Compassion	38.4	35.0	43.3	46.7
Professionalism	19.8	17.5	16.7	33.4
Efficiency	10.5	15.0	6.7	6.7
Accuracy	7.0	12.5	3.3	6.7
Privacy	3.5	5.0	3.3	3.1

Patients were able to identify more than one area, so totals exceed 100%.

Staff's Friendliness

In addition, "friendliness of staff" takes on additional importance, particularly for younger patients. One recent clinic patient summed up these feelings effectively: "People need to be treated as people, other human beings; not insurance claims. And being left for hours in waiting rooms is just unacceptable."

What the Results Reveal

We wondered what characteristics of customer service were the most likely to cause a strong reaction, good or bad. We asked patients to relate the best and worst example of customer service, and then we looked for common elements. Table 5.8 provides some insight indicating the most common "worst" experience.

Once again, "wait time" is at the top of the list. How often does a patient's contact with a hospital or clinic begin

TABLE 5.8

Patients' Most Common Complaints in Their Hospital Experience

Worst Examples	National Average	Older Patients (over 55)	Middle-Aged Patients (36 to 55)	Younger Patients (under 35)
Excessive wait times	40.8%	28.6%	52.4%	64.7%
Lack of professionalism	28.9	40.0	19.1	5.9
Not enough communication	26.3	28.6	33.3	17.7
Lack of compassion	25.0	20.0	33.3	23.5

Patients were able to identify more than one area, so totals exceed 100%.

with a long wait in registration, an examination room, or diagnostic staging area? "I was in the emergency room after having almost severed two of my fingers and waited for over an hour. Finally, I ended up going to another hospital, and they took care of me right away."

Patients are telling us that efforts to reduce healthcare costs are unacceptable if they have resulted in extensive staff and service reductions without making necessary operational adjustments or improvements in technology. Patients also expect professional, effective support operations and will not accept less: "I wasn't billed until 11 months after a brief hospital procedure. Even though I was upset, I mailed a check. But then they didn't record the payment, so I had to go in and 'fix' the situation in person. The hospital I go to now doesn't have those kinds of problems."

But what are the most likely things to cause a positive patient reaction? The answers, reported in Table 5.9, are more fundamental than you might think.

When combined, human compassion (47.1 percent) and friendliness (38.2 percent) were the key aspects of the "best"

TABLE 5.9

Patients' Best Experiences in a Hospital Related to Customer Service

Best Examples	National Average	Older Patients (over 55)	Middle-Aged Patients (36 to 55)	Younger Patients (under 35)
A showing of compassion	47.1%	42.9%	59.1%	36.4%
Friendliness by staff	38.3	37.1	36.4	23.4
Professionalism	26.5	31.4	27.3	9.1
Communication	25.0	11.4	40.9	16.4
Shorter wait time	23.5	14.3	27.4	45.5

Patients were able to identify more than one area, so totals exceed 100%.

customer service experiences in 95 percent of the respondents' comments. The solution almost sounds too obvious. "When I had to have an MRI, I was very frightened. The technician talked me through the procedure and kept encouraging me and talking to me so I would know someone was with me. It made all the difference in the world." "I will never forget one very special RN. She brought me a much needed box of Kleenex and gave me a hug while my husband was in a treatment room. He died recently of cancer, and that was one of my 'low days.' "

KEY FACTORS IN HEALTHCARE CUSTOMER SATISFACTION

So what are the key factors in customer satisfaction? We think patients have made their opinion clear. We broke their responses down into three categories:

- **Compassionate, friendly, and committed staff with excellent communication skills.**
  The most unique characteristic of any healthcare institution is its team of professionals—physicians,

nurses, and nonmedical staff. The quality of care they provide, as well as their ability to work together, will create the longest-lasting impressions of customer service in the patient's mind. Unfortunately, this is no small feat. Healthcare professionals are under great stress at many facilities. Most are ill equipped to handle the additional pressures of shrinking resources, aging facilities, and uptight co-workers. The foundation of any customer service improvement program appears to be a compassionate, upbeat, committed, and motivated staff trained in human relations.

- **Professional and high-quality services, provided efficiently, at hours convenient to modern work schedules.**

  In our consulting practice, we have repeatedly identified the cause of "extended wait time" as inefficient scheduling of procedures and ineffective admission procedures. Emergency rooms and other waiting rooms are all too often "clogged" with patients seeking nonurgent healthcare, because they can't access services during conventional schedules. Many hospitals have far too many patient processes that take patients from one waiting area to another with unnecessary long delays in each. Extended wait times can be fixed, and have been, at many healthcare facilities. If the patient (the customer) wants service during times at which providers currently do not provide them, providers should consider changing their schedule.

- **Adequate information, provided in a timely fashion, in understandable terms.**

  Patients want an explanation of procedures and medications. They want thorough instructions when they are discharged. They want to know about their treatment program. They want a bill they can understand and someone to explain the charges to them. Patients want healthcare providers to take the time to talk to them, listen to their concerns, and then provide them with information they can understand. These needs are too often not being met by providers today.

A recent editorial in *Modern Healthcare* put it this way:

> Wake up, Mr. and Mrs. Administrator. As an industry, healthcare just doesn't get it. Jack West, chairman of the American Society for Quality Control, put it best: "Quality is not what the quality professional says it is. It's not what the engineer says it is. It's what the customer says it is."[1]

---

1. *Modern Healthcare,* December 19–26, 1994, p. 38.

6

CHAPTER

Indifference Causes Its Own Kind of Pain

The words themselves are enough to make us stop, step back, and pause: *Blood. Pain. Fear of the unknown. Surgery. Anesthesia. Long, drawn-out illness. Death.* These are powerful words and powerful images too, images most of us would rather not think about for ourselves and for our loved ones. But no matter how much we close our eyes, close our hearts, and close our minds to those powerful and frightening words, the sad reality is that we all must face pain, illness, and death at some point in our lives. And someone, somewhere, right now, is facing it, even as you read these words. Maybe it's your mother or father. Maybe it's someone you know from work or someone who lives down the street. Maybe it's a total stranger, but someone is experiencing those things right now. Someone in a white paper gown walks down a long, lonely corridor. Meanwhile, a man clutches the hand of his wife of 40 years, watching for movement behind the eyes that will never again slip open and never again smile to see his face.

A skinny 12-year-old boy waits quietly to start his chemotherapy, a stuffed toy under his arm and a baseball cap pulled over his pale, bald head.

A young mother weeps for joy as she cradles her hungry daughter, only six hours old, against her breast, and her proud husband's hands shake as he steadies the camera, ready to immortalize the moment forever.

Two teenage boys sit quietly in the waiting room, grim-faced and firm as they wait to hear the results of their father's biopsy.

A middle-aged woman brings a bunch of pink roses for her elderly mother who, stricken with Alzheimer's disease, no longer recognizes the child she raised, but thanks her anyway, and inwardly marvels at the kindness of strangers.

A young woman on her knees in the hospital chapel prays fervently for her three-year-old niece, struck by a hit-and-run driver now entering her eighth hour of surgery.

These are our stories; yours, mine, and everyone's. Many of us have been there and all of us will all be there again, racked with worry, pacing the waiting room floors waiting for news about our mother. Or father. Daughter. Son. Sister. Husband. Friend. But if we are lucky, we will look up and find a kind face there to greet us, a warm smile and a pat on the shoulder, a few soft words of comfort and encouragement. It may be a busy doctor who takes time to explain exactly what went wrong, shows us the X-rays, and tells our loved one what to expect in the next few hours. It may be the head nurse who offers a tissue to dry those tears and a squeeze of the hand to let you know you're not alone. It may be the lab technician, who, instead of pointing to the cafeteria and saying, "Down there," takes our arm and walks with us, steadying our trembling steps along the way. A hospital can be a sad, scary, lonely place to many patients, but much less so when staffed by people who care. And that, ultimately, is what the customer service revolution in healthcare is all about: putting the human touch back into the healthcare system; restoring compassion to its rightful place at the start of the medical equation.

In purely clinical terms, the United States leads the world in medical miracles. Diseases once considered incommutable death sentences—tuberculosis, diabetes, leukemia, breast cancer, and kidney failure—can now be successfully treated, and in some cases, even cured. Procedures that formerly would have been considered the stuff of science fiction are now so commonplace that we don't even notice when we meet someone who has had a lung removed, a heart transplanted, or given birth through artificial insemination. We have become somewhat over-confident about our nation's medical potential, expecting that nearly everything in the human body that can break down can be fixed or replaced. The United States is the envy of the world in this respect, and patients travel from all over the world to seek treatments and cures at our world-renowned hospitals and institutions.

THE HUMAN ELEMENT HAS BEEN LOST

But there is, of course, a downside to our amazing achievements in medical progress. Somewhere along the line, the human element has become lost or forgotten. Or perhaps it was only misplaced, its luster tarnished among the gleam of all the ventilators, the vaccines, the dialysis, and the heart-lung machines.

The medical community has also become overconfident, even arrogant, in its assertion that it can treat any ill. Medical personnel are often accused of acting as if they themselves had the power of life and death. They often take on the arrogance of some celestial deity. It seems as if the entire medical profession has adopted a superiority complex about all facets of the delivery of healthcare in this country. Staff have gotten so good at saving lives, putting people back together again, and healing that the little niceties of life such as acts of kindness, thoughtfulness, and going above and beyond normal procedures are somehow beneath the personnel. Sometimes you get the feeling if the staff of hospitals and physicians' offices displayed acts of charity and compassion they would betray some medical oath of their profession. Indifference by those with whom the public comes in contact has become what patients have come to expect. A patient's physical well-being is the bottom line, indeed has become the only concern, and the only means of measuring success. A patient's mental, emotional, and psychological well-being all take a back seat.

Nearly everybody has at least one personal horror story to share; an example of professionals' behavior that goes beyond indifference to that of rudeness, insensitivity, blatant unconcern, or even medical malpractice. Such behavior results from the medical community's failure to *put the patient first*. Through our 1995 surveys and interviews, we talked to nearly 2,000 former patients about their healthcare experiences. Following are just a few brief examples of some of the more disturbing stories told to us by ordinary Americans, people who could be your family, coworkers, or friends, or patients.

A chief of nursing at his own hospital, Bill York of South Springs, South Dakota, told us of a humiliating experience with his pregnant wife:

> My wife, also a registered nurse, and I had preadmitted her and completed a "dry run" prior to her going into labor with our daughter. We were told to go to the emergency department of the hospital and ask for a wheelchair and an escort to labor and delivery. On arriving in the emergency department, no one even could find a wheelchair in the area. We were also rudely greeted by a male RN who asked, actually shouted at us, in front of the entire ED waiting room, "Honey, has your water broke yet?" I was so upset, I wrote the V.P. of nursing,

complimenting the labor and delivery care and recounting the above situation, but I never even received a response.

An elderly man from Alabama described how a lack of compassion by the hospital staff led him to digust:

> They let me lie on bloody sheets, with blood all over my pajama top, to the point that it had dried on my skin. Now if someone had checked on me during the night, they might have seen this. I had in two IVs and was unable to get the pajama top off by myself. In postsurgery, they plopped me in the bed and did not take my vitals for 55 minutes. They said they were "busy." If it had not been for my family who stayed with me, I might not even be talking to you now.

A 40-year-old woman from Kailua, Hawaii, reported how the rudeness of a physician's office staff could have had disastrous implications:

> When the doctor was confronted with several mistakes made by the office staff (waiting days to report vital lab results to patient, etc.), the doctor responded, "Well, you can go somewhere else if you want to." One other very bad memory I have is the physician's response at another facility a couple of years ago. When I suspected my child had Down's Syndrome (she did), right after delivery at 9 PM, the OB/gyne told me to wait until morning to have a pediatrician check her out! Luckily I insisted that my pediatrician be called, because a heart defect surfaced soon after and the baby was transferred to NICU at another facility within hours.

As disturbing as these stories sound, the most concerning aspect may be that these situations do not appear to be isolated incidents. Examples such as these appear to be all too common at hospitals and clinics around the country. One man who knows how widespread this kind of treatment is, Dave Gorden, is a Tennessee businessman and professional "mystery patient," whose undercover experiences as a patient in 49 different hospitals during the past 11 years have given him a unique insight into the state of healthcare services and patient satisfaction. The most significant thing that his experiences have taught him is that a little compassion can go a long way.

> In the hospital, you're a prisoner. I like to say that they give you a private room and a public gown. And they take control away from you. They tell you if you can go to the bathroom, when you can go to the bathroom, and what to do with it after you go to the bathroom. So when someone is kind, in what you and I, in a day-to-day situation might think is no big deal, in a hospital setting, it really makes a big impression.

HAIR-RAISING EXPERIENCES

As a mystery patient, Gorden has had his share of hair-raising experiences. At one hospital, where Gorden was under observation after pretending to have suffered chest pains, the phlebotomist had trouble drawing blood from his vein, so she decided to take it from his finger. She was in the process of doing that when an EKG technician came in to perform a test, which made the phlebotomist nervous. She proceeded to squeeze two vials of blood out of Gorden's finger, which he found quite painful. When she finished with the second vial, she started looking around because she had misplaced the first vial. The EKG technician helped her look for the vial, as did Gorden, who climbed out of bed with his IV still attached because, as he says, "I didn't want to go through this again."

The three of them looked everywhere and could not locate the vial, so the technician said, "It must be in the sharps disposal unit, in a locked box on the wall." The phlebotomist got the key to the box from the nurses' station, opened the box, and proceeded to dump the contents into the sink in the patients' bathroom. She said she found a vial of blood, which may have been the one she misplaced, but could easily have been somebody else's. The phlebotomist took that vial away and never came back to clean up the mess in the bathroom. Gorden tried to clean it up but worried about possible HIV contamination from the used needles among the refuse left in the sink. "I didn't know what to do," he admits. "That was the closest I ever came to calling the hospital administrator at home and saying, 'I'm out of here.' "

Several times Gorden has been a patient in a hospital for three or four days and never had a bracelet put on his wrist, which means the doctors and nurses didn't know whether they had the right patient for blood work, tests, and so on. Many times he has been presented with the incorrect medication. For example, he was once given a pill which is given to nonbreast-feeding new mothers to dry up their milk supply. "I didn't take it because I challenged the nurse and said, 'What is this?' And she went out and came back and said, 'Oh, I think that wasn't really meant for you,' " Gorden says. The result: The hospital still charged him $42 for that pill.

So what do patients really want from their healthcare providers? Are their expectations too high? Do they unreasonably expect the Ritz Carlton treatment from people who are often overworked, stressed, and in trying situations? Are they asking doctors, nurses, and technicians to go above and beyond the call of duty? Our research suggests not. The patient survey we conducted revealed that although customer service is extremely important to them, patients expect a 9.4 rating on an index scale where 10 is highest. The most important issues to patients revolve around simple, basic concepts like waiting time, privacy, and compassion. Following are some of the features of care that patients told us they want from their healthcare providers:

> "As a paying customer, I expect prompt, professional attention regarding my procedure, with a full understanding of what is going to be performed."

"No one wants to be neglected, ignored, or wait for unreasonable lengths of time."

"Familiarity with your insurance; no blame for the type of insurance you have."

"Patience and warmth."

"I want them to listen to my problem."

"Respect! To be treated as timely as possible, and with a friendly atmosphere."

"Explanation and discussion of treatment, symptoms, future expectations."

"Quick and still caring."

PATIENTS' EXPECTATIONS NOT UNREALISTIC

These issues hardly sound like unrealistic or unreasonable expectations. They reflect the level of service you would expect in a department store, a restaurant, or a car repair shop. Is it too much to ask for doctors, nurses, technicians, and other healthcare employees to supply the same level of customer service? Based on our research, the problems with customer service in healthcare can be divided into the four main areas that concern patients: communication, friendliness and warmth, compassion, and wait times.

Communication

A director of patient relations of a hospital in Albany, New York, told of how a lack of good communication by the hospital staff impacted his father:

> In October 1993 my father was a patient in a hospital in downstate New York. The staff—including nurses, physicians, nurse managers, and a VP—refused to answer his questions about his care. Even after I revealed my profession and my sister's, who is an attorney, the hospital refused to explain a nursing care plan, to tell us

why specific tests were ordered, or to tell my father what his diagnosis/prognosis was—and he's an alert and oriented 59-year-old! They stated that they have a patient representative on staff. It took me two days to find out that their patient representative is a volunteer who works on Thursday afternoons only!

A young mother from Graysville, Alabama, told us how a lack of communication caused her concern and pain:

> Having my first child by C-section after 17 hours of labor was exhausting and painful. Afterwards I was given a small amount of medicine and was told to, "Make it last, that's all you're getting." I lay there all night hurting until a new nurse took over and gave me the medicine I was supposed to get. I didn't know any better, I just accepted it . . . I think my first pregnancy and delivery were so bad that everything about the second one seemed better, even though I had another C-section after 14 hours . . . I also had a bad experience the second time, which was due to miscommunication between me and my doctor about the method of medication used after delivery. I ended up spending around three to four hours in tremendous pain. He thought he was saving me money. He did, but I paid for it differently.

Friendliness and Warmth

An elderly man from Lombard, Illinois, has bitter memories from his experiences in hospitals:

> The hospitals today are run by people with business degrees, with making a big dollar profit first instead of combining patient care with cost care. . . . My wife spent 75 days in a hospital in Arizona, 65 days of them in intensive care, and received a range of care from indifferent to bad. If I would not have been present, my wife could have died several times if I hadn't intervened.

A young woman from Nashville, Tennessee, described how she was treated for her weight problem:

I was treated as ignorant and fat. Most, if not all, of the information about my condition and my surgery was given to me in a handout in the hospital. I did not know what was in the future for my health until it was over. Please, please, inform doctors and hospital staff to treat their patients with respect. Tell them about the illness, the treatment, and the recovery.

Compassion

A 60-year-old woman from West Hartford, Connecticut, described how a lack of compassion by the hospital left her with bad memories:

> Being left unwashed for hours in a pool of blood after surgery. The aide was afraid to check the surgical area. . . . Having the nurse give me less pain medicine than ordered by the doctor. . . . Being very cold after surgery, both in the recovery room and on the floor, and having to wait a long time for someone to bring me a blanket.

A lack of simple compassion was often the complaint from patients we spoke with during the research. A 30-year-old mother from Oklahoma told us:

> Our one-year-old son choked on some popcorn. We did the Heimlich maneuver on him and he breathed again, but then little red spots broke out on his chest. We took him into the emergency room and we were scared to death. The nurse yelled at us, "Don't you know not to do this?" in a very rude way. We were so mad at her, we didn't care to ever return.

A man from Bisti, New Mexico, described an incident similar to ones we heard from many patients: "When I had a broken leg, the doctor just marched into my room and cut my stitches, then started cleaning my wound without telling me what he was doing."

The last days of her husband's life were characterized this way by a woman from Bloomfield, New Mexico:

My husband was very sick with acute leukemia and one of the nurses refused to do anything for my husband. I asked for service and she didn't come, so I reported her. My husband had a night nurse who wouldn't change him for his terrible rash. My husband died that week. He had such a poor nurse that night. I reported her. You wouldn't believe how much my husband suffered.

Wait Times

A retired Navy veteran voiced an often-heard complaint. "Much of the time patients get little time with the doctor, and the doctors are often quick to diagnose and slow to listen to the patient's questions and listen to the patient's answers. I've been a heart patient since 1984, and when I had emergency chest pains, many pertinent questions were not asked. The doctor left the unit to go home three hours early because he missed lunch. The doctor involved in reviewing and I assume, responsible overall, never saw me. Two weeks later he still had not yet advised me of the results. The charge for about 30 minutes was $3,900."

Although our research with patients uncovered some horror stories about customer service and patient *dis*satisfaction about practitioners within the healthcare field, the news is not all bleak. The American public has spoken. Patients are making their feelings known, through their employers and their managed care organizations. Slowly but surely, the customer service revolution has begun. Patients are demanding better services for their healthcare dollars, and hospitals and clinics have heard the alarm bells and are heeding their call.

PATIENTS DEFINE CUSTOMER SERVICE IN HEALTHCARE

As part of our patient satisfaction research, we asked the people we surveyed how they define the term *customer satisfaction* in healthcare. Their responses tell the story well:

"Customer service in a hospital means making the patient feel as relaxed as possible, and as comfortable, and letting the patient know that you're there to help him or her get well again."

"Be sensitive to your patients' needs, have empathy for patients' feelings of loss of control, confusion, illness, or pain. Customer service is based on understanding."

"Admitted quickly, procedures fully explained. People listened when questions were asked and showed support. Customer service is smiles, sincerity, patience, and support."

"A smile means the world to someone entering or leaving a hospital or doctor's office."

How simple and yet how profound; a smile, a hand-shake, a pat on the back. What do patients want? A reas-surance that yes, I am dealing with a fellow human being. For instance, Carrie Angus, a caregiver, says, "I got tired of being a pill-pusher." An internist by training, Angus faced a crossroad in her medical career. She decided on a less-traveled path that emphasizes a holistic/homeopathic approach to practicing medicine. Sometimes it's a smile or a touch, a look of concern, or the sound of doctor and patient laughing. However it is delivered, the message is clear. Angus cares deeply about people and helping them get well. She will hug them or rub their backs—anything to jump-start them on their way to wellness. "I treat them like they are my friends," she explains. "It enriches my life to be sincere. I couldn't do it any other way."[1]

Dave Gorden, the mystery patient we described earlier in this chapter, has had many positive hospital experiences as well as his horror stories. He has experienced the full, broad spectrum of treatment within hospitals, from horrific

---

1. *Milwaukee Journal / Sentinel.*

to wonderful. "I would say hospitals are, generally speaking, consistently inconsistent. When you are a patient, you are touched by 40 to 60 people a day, both directly and indirectly. You are directly touched by nurses, technicians, dietary, housekeeping, etc., and indirectly touched by the pharmacy, lab workers, food preparers, and others," he explains. This creates a broad potential for things to go right, or to go wrong:

> Nursing services may do a wonderful job, but the lab is slow in running the tests, or the phlebotomist is rude; therefore my overall impression of the hospital is affected. You can't average a hospital experience. That would be like standing with one foot in a bucket of ice water and one foot in a bucket of boiling hot water. On average, that wouldn't be very comfortable. When a patient is discharged from a hospital, especially after three or four days, they don't say, "The lab did a good job, the pharmacy did a good job, nursing was OK, dietary was not so terrific, and environmental services was lousy." That's not what they say. What they say is, "I had a miserable time in that hospital," and it's because one nurse didn't respond quickly enough to the call light, or some other such thing. I believe that it's imperative that every hospital discharge happy patients, because they don't ever tell the good stuff. But you miss one meal, or one thing's not right, or your medication doesn't come on time, and you go home and call folks long distance to tell them about it.

Gorden, in the guise of the mystery patient, does not go beyond asking for what any ordinary patient might request. He stresses that he does not go into the hospital as a "bad guy" trying to catch someone in the act of practicing bad customer service; rather, he tries to exemplify the needs and concerns of the "typical" patient and let the hospital staff respond accordingly. One example of a very good experience that he has had came at a certain hospital when he asked a volunteer for a copy of *USA Today*. The volunteer not only brought him the paper for free, but came to work 10 minutes early each day during Gorden's stay just to have time to pick up the paper and give it to Gorden personally, and still have time to get to her volunteer position without being late.

TRUE TEST OF PATIENT SATISFACTION LIES WITH PHYSICIAN

As important as management's role is in patient satisfaction, the true test of patient satisfaction is the interaction between doctor and patient, a thought echoed by leaders in the field. "The doctor-patient relationship is probably the single most important dimension of medical care," says sociologist Richard Frankel, director of the Center for Human Interaction at Highland Hospital in Rochester, New York.[2]

Consumer Reports magazine's comprehensive 1994 survey of 70,000 of its readers asked about their healthcare impressions and experiences. The results closely mirror our survey results from the summer of 1995. Both surveys found that the quality of communication between doctors and patients was perceived as a big problem. Respondents reported that their doctors were not open to answering questions, did not appear to listen to the patients' concerns, and didn't give their patients any advice on making healthy lifestyle choices or changes. The *Consumer Reports* study also found, alarmingly, that the patients of doctors who didn't communicate well were less likely to follow instructions and were overall less likely to take their medication or follow the proposed treatment plan, which in some cases lead to the continuation, or the worsening, of the patient's medical condition. This study crystallizes the issue: Good communication between doctor and patient is not just good

---

2. "How Is Your Doctor Treating You?" *Consumer Reports,* February 1995, p. 81.

business or some touchy-feely good PR issue; it can spell the difference between sickness and health. And in some cases it goes deeper even than that: a study published in 1994 in the *Archives of Internal Medicine* found that patients cited communication issues in 70 percent of malpractice depositions.[3]

This emphasis on good communication is a sentiment echoed by our survey respondents. One middle-aged woman from Alabama said it best. Customer service is "having the staff listen to your questions or complaints and also discussing your bill later. I equate customer service with communications."

BEING TREATED LIKE A HUMAN BEING, NOT JUST ANOTHER PATIENT

Our interviews yielded some feedback of good customer service and patient satisfaction that we share with you here as an encouragement, perhaps even as a beacon of light. Perhaps someday all patients will be able to echo the words of Richard Barnes of Empire, Alabama: "I was treated like a human being, not just another patient."

A 60-year-old woman reported, "I had excellent, smooth, emergency room care when I was admitted with a severe fracture. The doctor came quickly. I've had very smooth admissions and discharges on my previous two or three visits, including one-day surgery. I think that care in hospitals has improved greatly over the years. The service is much more organized, including admission and discharge, meal service, and all other supplies."

A patient's husband commented on a particularly caring nurse: "A nurse came from another station to comb my wife's hair after weeks of neglect. Another nurse who was not attending my wife went out of her way to wash my wife's hair, comb, and braid it for her. That's what I call caring."

---

3. Ibid., p. 83.

Some former patients remembered kindness:

"The emergency people were very kind and sympathetic to me and my concerns. They talked to me and calmed me down, all the time explaining to me what was going on."

"Most nurses are all attentive, kind, and helpful. Good nursing care is half the battle."

"At the hospital, even when we were left in a waiting room for a short time we were told, 'Your wait will be. . . .' The doctor answered all our questions and did not rush us out."

"The RN/receptionist who brought me a box of Kleenex and gave me a hug while my husband was in the treatment room."

"My care and treatment at the hospital was superior. My family and friends commented often on the compassion and exceptional care the staff exhibited. I have not stopped talking about the wonderful treatment I received and the efficiency of the hospital to my friends and business associates."

"In the time I was at the hospital I encountered many employees; janitorial, food services, doctors, technicians, etc., and no one was less than pleasant, helpful, and concerned about customers."

As many of these examples prove, the American public has become accustomed to the "medical miracles" and the never-ending medical advances with which this country has improved outcomes. However, they have never grown accustomed to the providers' indifference or cold, uncaring, rude treatment. They have griped about it for years to their neighbors, friends, and family members. Now their voice of displeasure is growing louder and being heard by those who will do something about it.

7

CHAPTER

Patient Satisfaction as a Low Priority for Most Providers

As we waded through our research on how hospitals are responding to patients' demands for improved customer service, I was reminded of an old story about Earl Weaver, the legendary manager of baseball's Baltimore Orioles. Weaver was known for his colorful remarks about the wisdom of various umpire's officiating calls, particularly if they were not favorable for the Orioles. One evening, Weaver was upset about what he believed was an inappropriate strike call. He placed himself inches from the umpire's face as he shouted: "Buddy, you're doing a lousy job tonight, and I sure as h--- hope you're going to get better. But I've got a sick feeling this may be as good as it gets."

We interviewed, visited, surveyed and analyzed dozens of hospitals and clinics of various sizes and specialties from all regions of the United States. Our objective was to determine what actions were being taken to improve customer service. We were on a mission to locate innovators and visionaries, and find examples of "prototype facilities." At one point in the process, all three of us were depressed by what we perceived to be a mediocre response by providers to this equivalent of a revolution in the healthcare marketplace. More than once, we wondered, "Is this as good as it gets?" However, we did find a few shining stars. Hospitals exist like Chapman General in Orange, California, which provides a level of customer service not unlike a fine hotel. Chapman General hired Debbie Firsker as the concierge manager and is modeling itself as the "Nordstrom's" of healthcare. She stated, "There is one person—that's me—designated to get to know all patients—visit with them every day—make sure their needs are met, and that's all I do."

Chapman General is a small facility, operating in a highly mature managed care market that has to differentiate itself to survive. It's not just surviving, it's flourishing.

We were awed by the attitude and commitment of the entire staff at Bradley Memorial, a 250-bed hospital in Cleveland, Tennessee. According to Lynn Dunlap, assistant administrator for nursing, things have never been the same since Dave Gorden was admitted in 1991 as a mystery patient. "I did not want our staff or physicians to think we were merely trying to catch things being done wrong. That was not our objective. Our objective was to lay the groundwork for changing the hospital's culture." And change they did. Today the culture of this facility makes it absolutely unique. Every employee, from the CEO, to the nursing staff, to the third shift housekeeper, is "engaged" in the Bradley guest relations philosophy.

We discovered that Holy Cross Hospital on Chicago's near south side took a unique approach to determine its patients' "wants" as they relate to customer service. The hospital's new management team wanted to improve hospitalwide patient satisfaction. The team looked at the whole organization and decided to develop specific standards of behavior for interacting with customers (both internal and external). To help the team determine the proper standards of behavior, members enlisted the help of customer focus groups. Using findings from the focus groups, the team defined a clear set of standards and expectations for interacting with customers. By articulating the standards and rewarding staff who consistently exceeded the expectations, the hospital found their "patient satisfaction" scores improving dramatically, and the facility has been able to sustain the improvement. Holy Cross recently was named one of the winners in the Hospitals & Health Networks and Coopers & Lybrand Fourth Annual Great Comebacks contest. Chicago Mayor Richard M. Daley also proclaimed July 22, 1994, "Holy Cross Hospital Day in Chicago."

CQI TO IMPROVE CUSTOMER SERVICE

Community Hospital of Anderson-Madison County in Anderson, Indiana, used the continuous quality improvement (CQI) process to improve their customer service.

Although this was an early CQI project, Community Hospital showed clearly how much a facility can accomplish by focusing on an issue and using many resources for problem-solving ideas. The hospital used data from Press-Ganey quarterly and special reports, interviews with selected patients, and consultations with other Press-Ganey client hospitals during their investigative process. By combining the information garnered through all of these channels, the hospital came up with several ideas for improving patient satisfaction with home care advice. Considering the changing focus in healthcare, the facility's decision to work on this issue was a timely one. The team realized that home care is of increasing importance to patients and their families and that to take care of the patient both in and out of the hospital, improved communication is essential. In the short time since implementation, patient satisfaction scores have gone up significantly.

St. Luke's-Roosevelt Hospital Center in New York City formed a patient relations group, the purpose of which was to find ways of improving patient satisfaction at the hospital. One of the group's many ideas was to create the Adopt-a-Floor program. Each unit was adopted by a physician and a member of the administrative staff. They formed (and worked closely with) a multidisciplinary team on each inpatient unit. The teams were charged with the mission of increasing patient satisfaction, resolving any problems that might arise, and improving the experience of being a patient. Each team continues to work to resolve the issues most important to that unit. The program has met with success as a result of the unit-specific solutions implemented by the teams.

Emergency rooms are hot spots for patient complaints in hospitals throughout the nation. Mercy Hospital Medical Center in Des Moines, Iowa, found a solution. Its busy emergency department (ED) noticed a dramatic dip in patient satisfaction as overcrowding became a serious issue. As staff frustration and patient complaints both increased, management made the bold decision to restructure the emergency department. The managers changed staffing patterns and rules regarding visitors. They also added space to the ED by moving some adjacent departments to other parts of the hospital, thereby making additional space available for the ED. They used the space to create separate areas for patients experiencing chest pain and for those needing "minor care." Since implementing these changes, Mercy Hospital has realized an increase in staff morale and has seen patient satisfaction climb.

A simple and effective approach taken by the Dannen-felser, Litwak, and Shasno Pediatric Clinic in Abingdon, Maryland, established a model for physicians groups that is built on developing a personal relationship with their patients' parents. The clinic established support groups for new parents, where complete information and answers to questions are provided by the medical staff. Emily Fleming, clinic administrator, summed up the approach, "We try to put ourselves in the mother or father's position . . . we try to understand it from their perspective. We try to treat them the same way we'd like to be treated."

MOST PROVIDERS DRAG THEIR FEET IN CUSTOMER SERVICE

We are convinced that intensified competition for patients covered under managed care plans has shocked a number of healthcare facilities into taking customer satisfaction more seriously. However, most are being dragged reluctantly into the new era of "customer friendly" healthcare.

It's disturbing to read the results of a University of Michigan research project designed to measure the quality of American goods and services. Surprisingly, the maligned manufacturing sector of the economy actually scored higher in a study of 46,000 customers than did service industries. The real scorcher was that on a 100-point satisfaction index, hospitals scored only a 74, somewhere between the 60 of the U.S. Postal Service and the 82 of long-distance telephone service.[1]

The good news is, this *is not* as good as it gets. The customer service revolution in healthcare is just underway. A few hospitals and clinics are developing innovative ways to "connect" with their customers. Facility managers are asking questions and listening to what the patient is saying. They are beginning to understand that if they don't adapt to meet the patient's needs, someone else will.

PROVIDERS HAVE TROUBLE IDENTIFYING "CUSTOMER"

If we've learned anything in our consulting practice, it's that sometimes asking the most obvious questions produces the most startling responses. That's what happened when

---

1. *Modern Healthcare,* December 19–26, 1994, p. 38.

we asked hospitals who their customer was. We thought the answer was obvious. As Table 7.1 reveals, it wasn't.

To say there was some confusion about this issue is to understate the passion with which the facilities responded. In fairness to the hospitals, many identified the patient as their primary customer but then went on to expound in great detail about how they also saw their customer as the medical staff, insurance companies, and employers. The medical staff was a recurring theme. Clearly, hospitals see the physician as their customer. Unfortunately, in the process, the patient's needs have too often been considered as a secondary issue. Undoubtedly, this is one reason the customer service revolution has taken hold: Patients have learned to harness the power of stating their expectations.

If ever there was evidence that many facilities just don't know who their customer is, it was provided by the 17 percent of respondents who told us it was "everyone." Most hospitals are trying to please everyone they encounter. This is a noble objective, but is it possible to achieve?

Facilities that have established a focused and successful customer satisfaction program have clearly identified the patient as their customer. James Killian, COO and executive vice president at Lake Forest Hospital in Lake

TABLE 7.1

Who Does a Hospital Consider to Be Its Customer?

Response	Hospital's Perceived Customers
39%	Patients and their families
20	Medical staff
17	Everyone
14	Employers
10	Third-party payers (insurance companies)

Forest, Illinois, summed up his facility's perspective, "We know that the patient is our customer, and we will do whatever it takes to meet and exceed their expectations. We actually provide patients with a guarantee. We'll go so far as to credit their account if they're not satisfied. Obviously, we can't guarantee the results of their medical treatment, but every other aspect of our service is included."

Bradley Memorial, a model for hospital guest relations programs, has the right approach. The facility exudes a culture in which all employees, volunteers, physicians, visitors, and patients are will be provided the finest personal care and surroundings. But all personnel are focused on the single objective of providing their guest—the patient—with the finest service possible.

Participating hospitals and clinics in our survey were queried as to whether they held a general consensus as to what constituted "the most important" factors in patient satisfaction. With the exception of patient wait times, we were somewhat surprised at how consistent their answers were with what patients had told us, as illustrated in Table 7.2.

TABLE 7.2

What Hospitals Believe Are the Most Important Characteristics of Customer Service

Response	Hospitals' Perceived Primary Customer Service Characteristics
55%	Compassionate staff with excellent communication skills
33	Professional high quality care and responsive staff
12	Choice of treatments, physician, facilities (including extra amenities)
6	Efficiency of operations, including minimal delays in service

WHAT PROVIDERS WILL DO TO IMPROVE
PATIENT SATISFACTION

The issue seems to be this: If providers know *what* is important in customer service, what will they do to *make it happen?* With the exception of the low priority hospitals afforded cutting down patient wait times, the facilities' managers were on target with what patients want. Most facilities seem to have an understanding of the importance of their human resources. Jane McManus, director of patient financial services at Tompkins Community Hospital in Ithaca, New York, stated that key staffing decisions were at the core of their patient satisfaction program. "Hiring the right people, in the right spots, particularly in registration and other 'up-front positions' is critical. Having customer-oriented people who have the ability to consistently smile and be personable with a real positive attitude has been a key to our success."

Glen Treml, vice president of finance at St. Agnes Hospital in Fond du Lac, Wisconsin, said that his CEO had established a hospitalwide philosophy of attentiveness to patient needs. "We found that as we improved operations, customer satisfaction improved. We also began to take the time to talk to our patients and listen to what they wanted."

Like Chapman General, St. Agnes operates in a highly competitive and fairly mature managed care environment. Even though the number of hospitals in Fond du Lac is limited, larger metropolitan markets like Milwaukee are only an hour or so away. Jim Sexton, CEO, summed it up, "Patients have more choices than we'd like to think. We've learned from experience that if we don't provide what they need, or if we make them angry in the process of providing their service, they'll go somewhere else. We can't afford to take customer service lightly."

The Role of the Patient Representative

One of the customer service initiatives that has been around a long time is the concept of a *patient representative*—one employee or an entire department that serves as a liaison between patient and staff, to make that link even stronger. Although this is often proven to be a very successful program, in some hospitals the patient advocate exists in name only. The mystery patient and customer service consultant, Dave Gorden, has learned this is often the case.

> Many hospitals have patient representatives. But if you were to ask, "Dave, do you think it's effective?" I would say, most of the time I think it's window dressing. If you represent that you have it and you really don't, you'd be better off not saying you had it in the first place. For example, if you put a card on the nightstand that says you have a patient representative on duty 24 hours a day, and then I call that number seven times and get no answer. That often happens.

In some hospitals, a patient representative is only available a certain number of hours a week. "That would be like saying, 'Oh yeah, we have a surgical suite, but it's only open on Thursday.' Well, then you're not a hospital," Gorden says.

ANOTHER OVERNIGHT SENSATION?

At times during our research, we wondered if the "customer service revolution in healthcare" might just become the latest buzzword or "management trend of the month." Then we discovered another interesting perspective. Attention to customer service is not a new initiative for many of the industry's "innovators." As Table 7.3 indicates, almost a quarter of those we interviewed who are actively involved in a customer service improvement program have been active for over a decade.

TABLE 7.3

Years Hospital Involved in Customer Service Improvement Programs

Response	Length of Involvement
22%	More than 10 years
19	6 to 9 years
26	3 to 5 years
22	1 to 2 years
11	Less than 12 months

Florida Medical Center in Fort Lauderdale, Florida, pioneered the concept of a "Patient Satisfaction Improvement Group" back in the late 80s. The center established a formal patient complaint mechanism and continues to use patient service coordinators to conduct specialized surveys. This modified CQI team provides critical quality information to managers throughout the Fort Lauderdale facility. Attention to the specific needs of our older patient demographic is essential. In addition to the high concentration of elderly patients, Florida hospitals work with many transient middle-income patients. To complete the picture, Florida has been a battleground for managed care contractors and complicated Medicaid regulations.

The revolution has continued to pick up steam as hospitals have gotten involved in the quality improvement initiatives of the Joint Commission on Accreditation of Healthcare Organizations (JCAHO). Many of the facilities we interviewed identified customer service objectives in conjunction with CQI and total quality management (TQM) initiatives in the early 90s. The JCAHO has recently added additional customer/patient service standards to its review process. The standards explain that these services are designed to respond to patient and family needs. The examples of implementation are as follows: a concurrent and retrospective survey of patient satisfaction is conducted.

Patients are asked questions about the hospital's performance through telephone interviews, questionnaires, or interviews. The hospital reviews the information it collected in relation to its major clinical care activities and support functions. In particular, dimensions of performance—appropriateness, availability, continuity, effectiveness, efficiency, safety, and timeliness of services—are reviewed. Based on the results of the reviews, the hospital refocuses its services or redesigns the existing process of providing services, as appropriate.

The scoring of this standard indicates whether or not the hospital's planning process considers the needs, expectations, and satisfaction of patients and their families and adjusts the plan for services accordingly.[2]

SO WHAT *ARE* HOSPITALS DOING?

The hospitals we surveyed were asked to identify their primary customer service programs. We grouped their response activities into six major categories, shown in Table 7.4.

TABLE 7.4

What Hospitals Are Doing

Program Type	Facilities Using Approach
1. Survey patients by mail or phone	56%
2. Customer service training programs	32
3. Focus groups	16
4. Process improvement to reduce wait time	16
5. Special department of patient reps	16
6. Patient focused care restructuring	14

2. Source of this information is *1996 Comprehensive Accreditation Manual for Hospitals.*

Patient Satisfaction Surveys and Focus Groups

Within the broad realm of surveys and focus groups, we have included all types of customer inquiry/interview programs. This includes telephone surveys, patient focus groups, and other patient contact activities. Although virtually all facilities have implemented some form of hospitalwide patient satisfaction survey, 72 percent of the hospitals we reviewed have implemented specialized programs that focus on particular service lines, or include patients in "focus groups." These focus groups consist of former patients invited together as a group to provide personalized feedback to the hospital.

The most common survey method used appears to be mailback surveys, although telephone and computer-based assessment tools are gaining popularity. There seems to be little uniformity in distribution methods. Some hospitals place reply cards in the service areas being reviewed; others send questionnaires out to patients 3-to-30 days after discharge. But a number of facilities have come up with unique ways to use customer surveys to resolve specific concerns or problems.

Brandywine Hospital and Trauma Center, a 208-bed hospital in Coatesville, Pennsylvania, is a good example. Faced with three seemingly competing objectives—increase collections, reduce collection expense, and improve patient satisfaction—Joseph Mannion, director of patient accounts, decided to develop a proactive customer service program. Patients were contacted by telephone immediately after they received their first statement. The sole objective of this call was to offer to answer any questions patients might have about their bill and identify any potential errors or inaccuracies in registration and billing information. Although some patients received additional follow-up calls, at no time was any patient asked to pay.

In addition to identifying and resolving problems with the hospital's billing system, Mannion got a bonus. Through extensive control testing, the hospital discovered it had improved patient satisfaction levels, as well achieving a significant increase in prompt patient collections.

Another example of using patient surveys was found at the Albert Einstein Medical Center, Philadelphia, Pennsylvania. Management's commitment to gather patient satisfaction results led to a concerted effort to solicit patient feedback. Members of the management team of the center were asked to call one patient daily to request their opinions. At the same time, the team saw responses to patient satisfaction questionnaires increase.

Clinton Memorial Hospital in Wilmington, Ohio, used a "patient satisfaction tool" as a measurement to improve quality. A significant cultural shift is usually required in any organization that implements CQI, and Clinton Memorial Hospital was no different. The hospital's director of customer services enlisted the help of the hospital's president and other managers to communicate the importance of improving services at the hospital. Together they worked to keep staff motivated and to prevent complacency when survey results demonstrated above-average customer satisfaction. Their dedication and foresight led them in the right direction, as they passed their JCAHO survey under the new standards with flying colors.

At Saint Joseph's Hospital of Atlanta, improving customer satisfaction is one of the goals in the 356-bed facility's strategic plan. It's also part of the hospital's employee incentive plan. Over the past four years, Saint Joseph's has conducted various patient, employee, community, and medical staff surveys. But, unlike many hospitals that conduct surveys and then shelve the results, Saint Joseph's uses the information contained in such reviews to set goals for positive change. To coordinate surveys and to improve accuracy, four years ago Saint Joseph's switched from written surveys to telephone surveys conducted by the Gallup Organization.

Gallup's sophisticated statistical analysis of data allows Saint Joseph's to identify areas that make a difference in a patient's hospital experience.

Patient-Centered Care: Asking Patients about Their Needs

Patient-centered care means more than just being nice to patients. It requires the development of patient care programs that meet patient needs as patients perceive them, not as professionals or hospitals do. The Picker/Commonwealth Institute has developed a patient survey instrument that allows patients to go beyond *rating* their care to *reporting about* their care. "The emphasis is not on the technical aspects of care but on whether the patient received the attention he or she felt was needed," according to Margaret Gerteis, program coordinator. Thomas Moloney, vice president of the Picker Institute's Commonwealth Fund points out, "Assuming good technology and good doctors, more patients are basing their choice (of a hospital) on what they can understand, which are mainly substantial differences in personal service."

So by definition, any hospital actively pursuing a patient-focused care program should also have in place a compatible patient satisfaction survey instrument. Improved patient satisfaction is the foundation of a patient-centered program for 124-bed Pomerado Hospital in Poway, California, a suburb of San Diego. Staff call the program "Patient First." The hospital received the 1994 Marriott Service Excellence first place award.

Modern Healthcare and Marriott Health Care Services sponsor these annual awards to reward programs that exhibit innovation in patient service, teamwork, and cost efficiency. The backbone of the first phase of Pomerado Hospital's project, Patient First, was the creation of a new

---

3. *Modern Healthcare*, July 18, 1994, p. 32.

position called "administrative partner." Improved patient satisfaction is the cornerstone of the program. It takes patients an average of 5.4 minutes to proceed from arrival to bed assignment, which is down from a minimum of 15 minutes. Patients now go directly to the appropriate nursing floor when they arrive at the hospital. An administrative partner greets them at the elevator and takes them to their room where the registration process takes place. A mobile wireless phone system allows administrative partners to be in continuous contact.

The Queen's Medical Center in Honolulu, Hawaii, has actively used patient focus groups to identify patient needs and monitor satisfaction levels. Lindsey Carry, director of patient relations, reported that the program was facilitated by a private research company and identified 25 "quality indicators." The research was validated through a telephone follow-up survey of 450 patients, and the indicators are now used on an ongoing basis to monitor performance throughout the hospital. Results are communicated to all levels, and a Performance Improvement Team dedicated to improving patient satisfaction has been set up to develop action plans based on their research.

It's Not Enough to Ask What I Want; You've Got to *Do* Something

The problem with sophisticated survey programs and focus group structures is that it is fairly easy to lose track of your original objective. We get so wrapped up in collecting data and ensuring data integrity that we forget why we asked the question in the first place. The objective starts to become more one of analyzing information and explaining variations than improving customer service. So we asked our provider respondents one more question about the survey process; what they do with the survey data. Table 7.5 summarizes their responses.

TABLE 7.5

What Hospitals Do with Survey Data

Responses	Action Taken
36%	Route to department heads
21	Route to quality committee
12	Route to "everyone"
12	Route to CEO
3	Route to marketing
85	**Route to someone**
6	Determine "plan of action"
6	Set and/or monitor performance targets
3	Post on the bulletin board

The hospitals' responses speak for themselves. Most of the institutions we talked to are primarily "routing" quality information around the hospital. In some facilities, it's an accountability issue. Everyone is interested in patient satisfaction, but too often no one has primary responsibility for ensuring it. We asked survey "guru" Irwin Press, PhD and cofounder of Press-Ganey, Inc., why so many hospitals don't seem to act on the data they collect. "It has everything to do with management philosophy. Survey data should not be used to discipline or rank one department against another. We encourage our clients not to focus on raw scores, but to identify and reward improvement trends."

Press believes that it's essential that hospitals *find out* where they can improve, then take action. But he points out that providers have to be willing to acknowledge their shortcomings. "Survey data is meaningless unless you use it, and when you use it, you can make a difference."

Determining the customer service problem or patient complaint and doing something about it has more than one ramification for hospitals. The JCAHO's *1994 Accreditation Manual* requires hospitals to improve performance. One of nine measurements of performance is patient satisfaction. Also, The National Committee for Quality Assurance development of the Health Plan Employer Data and Information Set (HEDIS) includes patient-satisfaction components in its 60 measurements. HEDIS is designed to help consumers and employers compare the performance of managed-care plans. Some 21 major HMOs—including Kaiser Permanente, Prudential Health Care System, TakeCare, and U.S. Healthcare—plan to use HEDIS to standardize consumer health information on satisfaction. Combined, they have 9.6 million enrollees, or 20 percent of the nation's total.[4]

Achieving Hospitalwide Buy-in to Patient Satisfaction Data

Many hospitals find that getting all departments to appreciate the full value of patient satisfaction data is somewhat difficult. Pennsylvania Hospital in Philadelphia, Pennsylvania, was no different. The marketing department and patient, guest and volunteer services teamed up to help other departments understand the data and make it work for them. To do this, they presented inservices with various departments periodically to review the data and to explain its value. Within months, the other departments began using the data and advanced to rapidly that they even began requesting more sophisticated analyses. As a result of the efforts by these two departments, the hospital is now getting more value from its reports.

Sinai Hospital of Detroit, Michigan, has made patient satisfaction a primary concern for the entire hospital. To encourage staff participation and acceptance of patient satisfaction as an important part of the services provided,

---

4. Ibid., p. 30.

the hospital has taken a number of steps. Managers reward staff who are mentioned favorably on patient surveys and recognize units that perform well. Their commitment has paid off in terms of greater patient satisfaction and lower costs.

Almost a third of the hospitals said they used employee education as their primary method of improving customer satisfaction. Training spanned a wide range of topics, from basic job skills to human relations and team building concepts. Albert Einstein Medical Center in Philadelphia, Pennsylvania, uses an institutional "values" program instituted in the early 90s to train staff to deal better with patients and each other. The program is mandatory for all employees, from the top to the lowest level.

Once again, Bradley Memorial Hospital in Cleveland, Tennessee, "set the pace" as it unveiled a comprehensive management training program in October 1994 referred to as "Bradley University." The curriculum is quite extensive, featuring 7 core courses and 11 management courses, but the customer service theme is woven throughout each class.

Effective training and education programs need to be focused, but should not be conducted only for a select group of managers, supervisors, and key employees. Our research indicated that the entire staff benefits from improved human relations, communications, and team building skills. In addition to improving day-to-day operations, each program made a notable positive impact on employee morale.

Specific Patient Satisfaction Programs

A number of innovative programs are designed to meet specific issues identified through surveys, patient interviews, and focus groups. The most effective are often the result of a hospitalwide, CEO-led initiative. Mineral Area Regional Medical Center in Farmington, Missouri, was facing increased competition from the major St. Louis healthcare providers. After the center's local competitor was acquired, the center's managers found themselves scrambling to differentiate themselves from the larger, more aggressive multihospital corporations.

The CEO immediately instituted hospitalwide meetings in which he communicated his vision of a "hospital without walls." He convinced the staff that they were in a superior position to service the needs of the community, because they were part of that community. He told them that by interacting with their friends, neighbors, co-workers, and associates, expressing concern for their needs (and when the opportunity presented itself, telling people about the hospital), the staff would market their facility more effectively than the billboards and TV ads purchased by their competitor.

Outside firms were brought in to bolster the center's marketing skills and provide human relations training for all employees. Consistent with the hospital-without-walls vision, Mineral Area Regional Medical Center instituted a community outreach program that involved major employers in their service area. The hospital went out to local employers' facilities and conducted free blood pressure and cholesterol screenings, in conjunction with preregistration informational sessions. The director of registration met with the various benefits administrators and communicated the value of facilitating the insurance verification process. After one year of "head-on" competition, the center has experienced little if any loss of market share. But the CEO reports that the positive impact on the staff has been even more satisfying. "We are truly a team, depending on each other's strengths, compensating for each other's weaknesses."

In an effort to achieve staff buy-in and emphasize the importance of patient satisfaction to an organization, St. Luke's Medical Center in Phoenix, Arizona, created a bit of healthy competition among nursing units. Department heads wanted to raise patient satisfaction with nursing overall, and they knew they needed staff buy-in to achieve it. They developed a series of "scoreboards" for display. The large, colorful, easy-to-read boards provided staff with the scores and relative standings at a glance. As a result of fun competition (including some good-natured wagering among department heads), staff have not just accepted the results, they look forward to each new report and the posting of their scores, and they are motivated to continue improving service.

In another example, the teamwork and dedication of staff and management at Wilmington Hospital, Wilmington, Delaware, skillfully created a more patient-satisfaction–oriented culture through the use of Press-Ganey's patient satisfaction surveys and results. Significant improvements were made in the areas of visitor and family issues, cheerfulness/decor in patient areas, diet/meals, information to patients, and overall emphasis on caring and courtesy in every interaction with patients and visitors. The improvements were based directly on patient and employee suggestions.

There are numerous other examples, some of which are detailed in the following case studies. But the most impressive common denominator was that someone inside each facility took action. The action was based on a deficiency identified by getting in closer touch with patients.

Facilities Improvement

As healthcare profit margins have declined in the last 10 years, hospital plant and equipment have suffered. Although most facilities have done a good job maintaining existing resources, many institutions have found themselves with buildings no longer suited to the current marketplace. As lengths of stay have declined and providers have shifted to more performing ambulatory, outpatient procedures, large inpatient "monuments" have become an unnecessary overhead expense creating a logistics nightmare. Providers have found themselves in the position of being "forced" to remodel and invest in new facilities. The patient-focused care concept that most often requires a restructuring of some or all of the patient floors was mentioned frequently by hospitals as a means to improve patient satisfaction.

Some of our respondents told us that their primary "customer service improvement program" included renovation of a specialty area or emergency department. The William Beaumont Medical Center in Royal Oak, Michigan, is a good example.

- Emergency departments are being expanded to provide for more immediate triage as well as 24-hour, nonurgent medical needs.
- A comprehensive women's center provides mammography, maternity, and other OB/gyne diagnostic procedures in a low-stress, high- service-level environment.
- The ambulatory surgery unit is freestanding and provides for easy access and immediate service.

Other facilities are expanding less dramatically, but with the same objective: to serve the patient more efficiently.

Perhaps most dramatic is the development of entirely new facilities, designed from the ground up to meet patients' needs. A good example is the Austin Diagnostic Medical Center that opened in Austin, Texas, in July 1995. In addition to inpatient diagnostic procedures, it is designed to handle more than 15,000 outpatients per month. The center established customer satisfaction/patient satisfaction as its primary goal. According to Charles Pearce, the medical center's chief operating officer, the facility intends to make customer service "more encompassing."

Patient service representatives will act as greeter/ hostesses to escort patients from arrival to bed. The same person will be there each weekday. Discharges will be prearranged using an integrated computer system. Reps will be "linked" to physician offices, and key information will be shared to better facilitate patient care. The "business side" of the hospital admission will be largely transparent to patients during their stay.

Starting from the ground up has its advantages. In preparation for their opening, the Austin Diagnostic Medical Center focused on identifying the best staff, then provided them with clear expectations on performance. Pearce thinks communication and staff training will be key to "making good" on his commitment of superior customer satisfaction.

The McCamy Hospital and Convalescent Center in McCamy, Texas, operates 16 acute and 30 long-term care beds, because they've listened closely to their community, and have adapted their operations to meet the community's needs. Dr. Ronald Freake, administrator for laboratory and home health services, told us that the facility has an active patient communication program, including an ongoing column in a local newspaper. According to Freake, "We're here to serve the community—period. But the way we accomplish that has changed. Once a hospital was simply supposed to provide medical services. Now, you've got to market those medical services or you won't survive."

Healthcare professionals in general need to understand that the patient is in fact their customer. Today, more than ever before, it's a competitive marketplace. Patients no longer have to go to a hospital for many medical procedures. Patients are much better educated now than before and react much more like consumers. Healthcare has become a consumable item.

CQI/Quality Teams

One of the best examples of a "customer service based" CQI/Quality team was headed up by Dave Albrecht, vice president of finance at Bellin Hospital in Green Bay, Wisconsin. Albrecht was attempting to merge two internal units (registration and patient accounts) that had not always seen eye to eye. "The managers from both areas were very dedicated but too often focused on their specific organizational responsibility. The challenge we faced was to harness their individual commitment and high standards in a way that better met the ultimate needs and desires of our patients," he said.

His strategy included site visits of facilities unrelated to healthcare that had similar "service" objectives. He focused on the financial and hospitality services industry. He believes this was a critical step: "We were able to 'step out of the conventional box' we'd placed ourselves in. By looking at other industries, we felt less ownership and defensiveness for the way it was always done," Albrecht recalled.

HOSPITALS' PLANNING: MORE OF THE SAME

If the customer service revolution has in fact just begun, it's reasonable to assume that healthcare providers will accelerate their improvement initiatives during coming months. That is not the case based on what our results showed. We asked respondents to provide us with a preview of their plans. The responses, listed in Table 7.6, showed that their contemplated actions are primarily a variation of what they are already doing.

Responses typically centered around conducting patient surveys, setting up focus groups, training staff in customer service techniques, and setting up special committees or task forces to address customer service issues. It appears that providers are planning on pretty much continuing their existing approaches with some fine tuning here and there. Repeatedly we recorded their response as, "Keep on with what we're doing," or "Nothing additional." The word *continue* came up in more than one-third of the hospitals we interviewed.

Many of the other responses in terms of facilities' plans for the future to improve patient satisfaction were new to them, but not to the industry, such as surveys, training, and

TABLE 7.6

What Hospitals Plan to Do to Improve Services

Responses	Activities Planned
40%	**Operational Programs** • Internal customer relations divisions such as patient representative departments • Reorganize and expedite registration functions • Institute "patient-focused care" applications • Evaluate and revise discharge planning and procedures • Customer service training for employees • Form special committees
33	**Surveys, Tracking, and Focus Groups** • Additional, more focused tracking and monitoring • Direct patient contact programs • Institute new patient focus groups
27	**New Equipment and Facilities Improvement** • New, expanded computer systems • Improved ERs, outpatient facilities

focus groups. Some additional alternatives were hiring a consultant; uniforms for the clerical staff; remodeling some of the units; creating "core" committees; going to the patient-focused care concept; and starting a concierge-type program.

In summary, our distinct impression from the 1995 study was that providers don't get the message about customer service. We sense they are not tuned into the movement toward the demand for improved medical services. Most providers do not seem to sense this customer service revolution on the horizon.

In our opinion, more of the same isn't enough. The demand for a higher level of patient satisfaction will mean providers must go far beyond their past actions. Patients have told providers that they want better customer service. Employers are now in the act and they will ensure that providers get the message. In short, those providers who score high by patients in the customer service issues will become the providers of choice in the managed care network. Those who score low will lose patients and revenue.

8

CHAPTER

Excellence through a Cultural Conversion

A Case Study: Bradley Memorial Hospital

There are numerous approaches to improve customer service by healthcare providers. None is more thorough and successful than what we witnessed at Bradley Memorial, a 251-bed hospital in Cleveland, Tennessee, serving a five-county region that offers a vast array of specialized medical, surgical, and diagnostic services through its more than 160 physicians, 1,000 employees, and 250 volunteers. Their service area has a total population of approximately 180,000. There are 15 hospitals operating in Bradley Memorial's service area with its primary competition located in nearby Chattanooga.

We have isolated Bradley Memorial to profile in a detailed case study because we felt this midsized hospital in a community of 80,000 located 30 miles north of Chattanooga exemplifies how customer service should work at its highest level. This facility not only excels at customer service but practically every other aspect of service that a hospital typifies or should typify in today's healthcare environment.

But first, let's consider customer service. The proof of the level of customer service always lies with patients' perceptions. Bradley Memorial ranks in the top half of all hospitals surveyed in overall patient satisfaction, based on the standard items in the Press-Ganey survey. Nursing service ranks in the top 14 percent of the nearly 500 hospitals whose patients are surveyed by Press-Ganey. Bradley's nursing department scored an excellent 91 out of a 100 index by their patients in the most current quarterly ratings. Service ranking doesn't get much better.

Based on other internal patient satisfaction measurements—such as hundreds of complimentary letters from their patients, their own patient satisfaction survey, and our interviews and talks with hospital employees as well as people in the community—Bradley comes across as an exceptional hospital that lives and breathes excellent customer service.

Dave Gorden, the healthcare guest excellence consultant working with Bradley who also consults for corporations including Hallmark, McDonald's and Walt Disney World, stated,

> In three years, this hospital has made incredible progress. You can feel it in the halls. Other hospitals come here and visit and say, "I don't know what it is about this place." I have a friend whose mother died in this hospital. Before she died, he told me, "There's something about this place." I said, "What is it?" He said, "People care. You walk through the halls and you feel people care."

CUSTOMER SERVICE PERSONIFIED

During our week-long, in-depth visit to Bradley Memorial, we witnessed the staff members' unique display of warmth and sincere caring attitude toward patients and toward each other. As we interviewed employees, roamed the patient floors, sat in waiting areas, ate in the cafeteria, and talked to the nursing staff, we experienced customer service personified.

But customer service is not the only area in which Bradley Memorial excels. In 1994, the hospital was selected one of the Top 100 Hospitals in America through the Benchmarks for Success study conducted jointly by HCIA Inc. and Mercer Health Care Provider Consulting. In 1995, the hospital received honorable mention. Bradley was one of only three Tennessee hospitals chosen in 1994. Only one Tennessee hospital was chosen as one of the Top 100 in 1995.

The dramatic announcement of the Top 100 in the faxed message that landed on the desk of Administrator Jim Whitlock at 5 PM one Friday aroused more skepticism at the time than excitement. "I thought it was a gimmick by a consulting firm," confesses Whitlock of the notification in January 1995 that Bradley Memorial had been chosen as one of the 100 top-performing hospitals in America. "I almost threw it in the garbage." It wouldn't have mattered; the award was for real. An official letter and description that arrived the following Monday named Bradley Memorial 1 of only 3 hospitals in Tennessee, 1 of only 19 hospitals in the South, and 1 of only 25 rural hospitals in America to make the exclusive list of 100.

Now, after accepting the prestigious award and after being recognized by peers, the community, and the media, the selection seems not at all surprising. For all along, Bradley has been sowing the seeds for unusual success. "We have an attitude of caring enthusiasm that permeates our organization, and that has to make a great hospital even better," beams Whitlock. "When you nurture this kind of spirit, it flows to the patient rooms and shows up in the indicators that measure the level of care."

Underlying the success by Bradley is the attitude staff members bring to their jobs each day. They seem to have employees who see beyond their job descriptions to the broader needs of the hospital. You can sense and see the value placed on teamwork, and the self-motivating sense of pride in what employees have developed. The basic measure of success or failure for any organization is individual attitude. The shaping of positive attitudes is an ongoing, high-priority process at Bradley.

In the midst of all of this, the hospital is in the middle of an ambitious multimillion dollar improvement plan. In 1993 the hospital embarked on the second and third phases of its 10-year expansion program. The $22 million construction project included development of an outpatient medical mall, a new women's center, a parking garage, education facilities including a public auditorium, advanced diagnostic imaging facilities, and a cardiopulmonary center. What is so striking is the fact the hospital embarks on the unusual to maintain their unique approach to customer service. For instance, the facility boasts its own hospital mascot and employees purposely try to catch one another doing something "beyond the demands of their job as it relates to customer satisfaction." Last year, they had their own parade down the streets of Cleveland.

In 1992, Bradley introduced the hospital's first mascot, to the community at the annual "Teddy Bear Clinic" hosted in the hospital's pediatric unit. The Teddy Bear Clinic, now in its seventh year, is designed to lessen the fear most children endure when told they need to go to the hospital. Employees set up a mock operating room where doctors, nurses, and other staff members perform surgery on stuffed animals. The volunteers sew up holes, fix fractures, bandage boo-boos, and even create limbs. For the sake of the children, they triage, admit, care for, and discharge their stuffed animals much like staff do daily for real patients. While their furry friends are in surgery, the children play games, win prizes, enjoy refreshments, and learn a great deal about the hospital and the people who might one day take care of them.

A HOSPITAL WITH ITS OWN MASCOT

The mascot for the hospital, *Brad Lee Bunny*, is a truly southern bunny named after the bunny's home county. Brad Lee was one of the hospital's strategies for making new friends and customers. Brad Lee lent the hospital a personality and identity, particularly in terms of the hospital's relationship with children. Brad Lee Bunny visits area schools, entertains at hospital events, participates in community sponsored parades and events, and appears at other select public events. Additionally, Brad Lee is featured in the hospital coloring book and serves as the focus of the Guest Excellence Get Caught promotion material and specialty items.

Somewhere along the way, the hospital developed a special program designed to "catch" employees and volunteers who exemplified the guest excellence philosophy by doing more than the daily demands of their job. Initially, the "catchers'" mission was to identify and catch employees and volunteers worthy of recognition. If caught, the individual was awarded a certificate that could be turned in for food in the hospital cafeteria or an item in the gift shop.

In order to keep the catcher program alive, the Guest Excellence Task Force changed the rewards, expanded the number of catchers, and enhanced the value of the rewards. Bunny Bucks, featuring the slogan "Get Caught" with the Guest Excellence logo, and Brad Lee Bunny were created. Bunny Bucks can be awarded by any catcher. The first time a person is caught he/she receives five Bunny Bucks and a Get Caught T-shirt. Each consecutive time someone is caught the ante goes up 10 Bunny Bucks, which can be spent in the hospital gift shop to buy specialty items such as baseball caps, umbrellas, tote bags, and coffee cups. Each person who is caught is eligible for a monthly cash drawing ($50) and every person caught is included in a drawing at the end of the year for a trip of their choice to the Smokey

Mountains, Panama City Beach, or Myrtle Beach. Approximately 60 people are caught each month by the 25-plus catchers representing numerous departments on all shifts. Each month on the front page of the hospital newsletter, "The Pulse," all caught persons are featured by name and department.

Bradley is also big on employee education and management development, with an overall view to also improve their customer service. Mickey Mouse has "Disney University." Ronald McDonald has "Hamburger University." And Bradley has Bradley University, a comprehensive management training program. Developed by the hospital's Guest Excellence Task Force during the past two years, Bradley University offers managers and aspiring managers the opportunity for professional and personal growth and development.

"To my knowledge no other hospital offers a program like Bradley University," Jim Whitlock told us. "We have committed the resources and time to our managers, and staff members who want to become managers. What they need to develop managerial skills is provided on-site on a regular basis and extends well beyond what most organizations would consider a training program."

The curriculum at Bradley University is extensive, featuring 7 core courses and 11 management courses. All courses are taught by members of the hospital staff who have either masters-level training or a bachelors degree and experience in the field of study for which they were selected as instructors. All hospital managers are required to attend Bradley University and must successfully complete all core courses within 6 months and all management courses within 18 months.

A FACILITY THAT CELEBRATES EVERYTHING

Staff celebrate everything at Bradley, from the traditional award banquets to each phase of the new building project.

When the hospital completed its first phase of construction, employees positioned a large balloon replica of a space shuttle on the canopy of the main patient tower facing the street signifying "space exploration." For the celebration, they had a cookout for employees and their families under a large circus tent on the hospital campus. Another special event was a black-tie, invitation-only program for donors, physicians, board members, political leaders, and other dignitaries. Held at night in the tent, the event attracted more than 250 people who were given the opportunity to have their photo taken with space aliens as they toured the new floors. An afternoon presentation for all members of the Cleveland/Bradley County Chamber of Commerce was held followed by an open house for the public.

When staff kicked off Phase II of the construction project in 1994, they knew there were mixed feelings among the staff members and former hospital employees about the demolition of the hospital's original 1952 wing. There was a strong sentimental attachment to this wing for those who had cared for patients on this unit. Through the magic of paint, wallpaper, costumes, and music, they took a make-believe step back in time. On the night of the celebration, staff and guests traveled back to 1952 when the hospital first opened. One room was transformed into a local cafe complete with jukebox, kitchen table, and soda fountain. In another room staff created a family living room circa 1952 with furnishings purchased from local shops specializing in vintage merchandise. The room was authentic down to the style of wallpaper and black and white television. Actors in vintage costumes circulated throughout the unit, talking to people about the hospital in its early days. Old photographs of the building and employees were available in scrapbooks and photo albums for all to review. Guests paid tribute to those employees from the past, something you seldom see nowadays.

During the new construction Bradley designed and built a new $1.4 million emergency center and reorganized the personnel in order to give better customer service. The facility even gave the center a new name: Super Department. The staff developed a new operational philosophy in ER in an attempt to create an environment where employees feel empowered to make decisions that affect the way services are provided.

The department was given four guest service ambassador positions whose primary functions include:

- Greeting guests in accordance with the hospital's Guest Excellence Creed and Philosophy when they enter the emergency center lobby.
- Notifying triage (evaluation) nurse of each new patient.
- Providing directions to patients and visitors searching for other hospital departments.
- Assisting persons who need help getting from the vehicle into the lobby.
- Monitoring the lobby for cleanliness and order.

Dressed in teal green blazers, white shirts/blouses, and either navy/khaki skirts or pants, the ambassadors try hard to exemplify the "Bradley image" in both appearance and action. The ER ambassadors are scheduled for three-hour shifts, seven days a week and are currently under the direction of the Super Department's administrative director.

Bradley also impacted the community with the formation of the Bradley Healthcare Foundation, created in 1991. It is composed of citizens of the community, and its primary purpose is to involve the community in a variety of ways, all designed to have a favorable impact on customer service.

CONNECTION BETWEEN PATIENT AND EMPLOYEE SATISFACTION

We have detailed many of the actions Bradley has taken during the past several years to convey the distinct impression that the facility is a successful provider where employees have fun on their jobs. And that's a key point to remember in making the connection between excellent customer service and employees enjoying their work. These employees do enjoy their jobs and have fun doing it. It pays off in the way they treat their customers, the patients. This success didn't just happen. Jim Whitlock worked long and hard over his five-year tenure as CEO at Bradley to develop a culture in which employees get a kick out of high performance regardless of their department.

The question that demands to be asked is, "How did this hospital reach this pinnacle of customer service and turned-on employees?" We'll attempt to answer that in the next few sections devoted to Bradley. We have chosen to illustrate Bradley because we feel its approach to customer service is one to be imitated by hospitals around the nation. If this model could become a prototype for other hospitals, not only would their customer service improve, so would their overall organizational management.

Dave Gorden, the guest excellence consultant, noted, "There is a hunger for what we're doing here. It's an exciting place. I've been a mystery patient 49 times now. I live 2 hours and 20 minutes from here, but if I can make it, this would be my hospital of choice of all the hospitals I have worked with the past 11 years. There are two or three hospitals that would be my last choice. I'd rather go to a veterinary clinic than go to one of those places. There's a big difference. It's come a long way in a short period of time because there's commitment and there's vision."

Bradley illustrates many of the traditional approaches toward customer service. The managers use the Press-Ganey surveys to follow up on complaints and to improve patient satisfaction. The facility created a special task force that comes up with ideas for customer service improvement and training programs aimed at improving employees' skills in customer service. Bradley invokes a variety of techniques to keep the customer service theme alive.

But Bradley's leaders go far beyond the traditional approaches. More importantly, they have changed the way employees *think* about their jobs. They have changed the way the employees think and act toward one another. They have changed the way the employees think about *their* hospital (and they truly feel it is *their* hospital). Leaders have managed to develop an entirely newmind set and culture at this hospital, one built around relationships. Relationships thrive among themselves, from top management through department heads, through supervisors and down to each staff member in each department. And, most importantly, relationships thrive with Bradley's patients. Customer service has become a "state of mind" at Bradley.

You won't find the real answer to improved customer service in patient survey surveillance, canned training programs on customer service, special departments set up to police customer service throughout the organization, or any other of the many and usually ineffective plugged-in approaches. What exists at Bradley are employees who practice excellent customer service because they feel it is the "right thing to do and they want to." In fact, staff seem not even to know they're performing some kind of customer process or procedure. They do what comes naturally. They care about each other and their patients. The caring is sincere and it shows.

That was not always the case at Bradley. The culture began to change when Jim Whitlock assumed the administrative reins in 1990 and began his cultural change. Everyone has come to call it a *culture conversion* because we liken it to a *spiritual conversion* that involves drastic change in *belief*. During the past five years this hospital incorporated a new belief system built on personal relationships, trust, believing in themselves, and believing in the role they play in their jobs.

Over the next three chapters, we will take you through this cultural conversion and the positive impact it had on Bradley's customer service. It is worth studying because the *conversion* can be emulated in most healthcare environments.

9

CHAPTER

Unleashing Customer Service through Servant Leadership

Customer service becomes a reality when employees in an organization virtually become permeated with an attitude of caring for the well-being of others. The key is in their attitude toward others. Their attitude reflects how the employees see themselves and the importance of their role in the success of the organization.

When employees view customer service as an inherent part of their performance, it becomes a natural act, not a "program" based on "technique" or reacting to patient grievances by running down patient survey complaints or nasty letters to the CEO. Good customer relations delivered by all employees all the time is more effective than an effort headed up by a special guest relations department in the hospital whose main task is often to police customer service throughout the organization. Customer service task forces, committees, and focus groups can only identify problems, analyze them, and create ideas to solve them. They cannot *implement* good customer service. Only the employees throughout the organization can actually make it happen day in and day out, month after month, year after year.

A powerful impact is generated in an organization when enough individuals are unified under a common cause such as commitment to customer service. A critical mass is built as individuals catch on to the idea. Soon it seems that more and more employees have the spark of customer service, and the idea spreads throughout the organization. It is at this point that employees question outdated processes and system limitations that everyone could always point to as an excuse for not doing better. Even employees who seemed unmovable in their resistance to change can be won over. Their laments of, "I've been here over 20 years and we've always had the same problems," and "We've been through this before and nothing ever changes," begin to fade when significant improvements are made. Winning resistors over only builds strength to the commitment.

How do managers achieve this employee attitude toward customer service throughout the organization? It starts at the top and works its way down through every department. But it must begin at the top, with the CEO, then to the rest of top executives, on to the department heads, supervisors, and then all the other employees. It begins with a management philosophy and a leadership style that creates openness, trust, and an environment in which employees know they have a voice in the decisions that impact their job. It begins with a CEO that possesses *servant leadership*. In Bradley's case, that person was Jim Whitlock, who joined the hospital as an assistant administrator before becoming the CEO in 1990. Now in his mid-50s, Whitlock cut his teeth on hospital administration with 17 years in the hard-nosed, bottom-line–oriented, for-profit chain of hospitals, Hospital Corporation of America.

However, Whitlock is anything but narrow-minded, hard-nosed, bottom-lined–oriented. He's proven to be firm and acutely tuned into the financial well-being of the hospital with his ability to make tough decisions when he has to and the fact that Bradley has been a highly profitable hospital in the past five years. However, he's much more than a professional at hospital finance. Whitlock's leadership style could best be described as subtle, participative, and patient with a strong, unyielding belief in his fellow human beings. Couple that with a large dose of optimism and the ability to visualize the future, and you might summarize his style as *servant leadership*.

TAKING SERVANT LEADERSHIP THROUGHOUT THE HOSPITAL

The key issue to address about leadership at Bradley is how Whitlock got his servant leadership mentality beyond himself and his senior staff and implemented throughout the entire hospital. It took several years. He started with his team of senior executives that reported to him. His first objective was to convert their attitude and thinking toward themselves and those who reported directly to them. Whitlock desperately wanted a more participative management style to permeate the organization to replace the stagnating and repugnant autocratic management approach that had prevailed at the hospital for nearly 40 years. Although he didn't know it at the time, his management philosophy and servant philosophy would pave the way for excellent customer service.

Jim stated that he began by developing a close relationship with his senior management team:

> The only thing that really changed in early 1990 was the fact that I was the new administrator and we seemed to meet a whole lot more. In retrospect, I think this was very important. I didn't say we agreed a whole lot more or worked a whole lot more or differently; we just met a whole lot more.

When he met with selected members of his senior staff, Whitlock had identified a core group of seven people: Michael Willis, Lynn Dunlap, Jeannie Roark (ex-controller), Dan

Cooper, Dan Gilbert Dewayne Belew, and Larry Ingram. With the exception of Dewayne Belew, all had preceded him at Bradley by at least four or five years. Although Dan Cooper was hired about the same time Whitlock joined Bradley, he knew there were at least three staff who didn't want him there, three who weren't sure, and one (Dewayne) that he could count on. He had some odds to overcome at senior staff level.

First, Whitlock recommended consistency. Every Tuesday morning senior staff would gather in a conference room at 8:00 AM. They had no agenda beyond what they wanted to discuss. From the beginning, Whitlock took the seat at the head of the table. "In retrospect, I think that was a good move. I considered an alternative position, but decided this gesture of authority was not only traditionally acceptable but was a nonverbal way of ensuring, for their security and peace of mind, that someone would always be there to protect them from themselves and each other."

Although other cumulative meetings were called on somewhat of an ad hoc basis, the Tuesday morning gathering was sacred. It would last four hours and frequently go beyond or even through lunch. It became the "tie that binds." To make it more informal, staff had breakfast served and the first 15 to 20 minutes were dedicated to socializing. Various staff members selected their positions and reported to them each week religiously. No one challenged their selection, but it was obvious to Whitlock that there were some hidden agendas along with a "pecking order" left over from the previous administration.

In retrospect, the benefit of this weekly gathering, unstructured as it was, was that it launched the long trek toward team building. Staff began to evaluate their specific roles and how they blended with each other. They began to "pick their friends" and confide in them outside the system. "I know they evaluated and speculated on my management style and personally, that is essential for an effective leader," Whitlock told us.

Dewayne Belew, the creative, high-energy, young director of marketing and public relations recalled his impression of the beginning of the team-building process under the new CEO.

> I wondered how much things were going to change. Although Jim had been here as associate administrator, he was now *the* Administrator. Right off the bat Jim started pulling the senior management team together as often as possible to discuss a variety of issues. Initially Jim was a strong advocate of Management By Objective and we followed this course of action. Eventually, we discovered that MBO was not the most effective management strategy for us. In all likelihood, we would not have discovered a management style unique to our team had we not committed to spending so much time together and valuing each other's input.

Belew was not sure anyone could calculate the number of hours they spent together in the south conference room on the first floor of the main tower. "The closest guess would be a gazillion hours." In this case, time together meant enhanced awareness of each other's personal style and professional strengths and weaknesses. Senior staff were able to identify the unique talents of their management group as a whole and as individuals. For them, the sum of the whole was truly greater than the parts. They jelled. The chemistry was right. There was synergy. "Any way you want to put it, we were able to bottle the magic," Belew recalled.

TUESDAY MORNING MEETINGS BECAME LEGENDARY

The Tuesday morning meetings, now legendary throughout the organization, still operate without a formal agenda four years later. Generally speaking, each manager creates his or her own agenda and presents each item for discussion and review when the staff circle the breakfast table.

For the first few months, the meeting was akin to wading into the water with no one wanting to jump in until he/she knew how deep it was. Each of them had things to discuss but needed time to gauge how far to go with each item. The team members came from different academic backgrounds, trained in various schools of management theory, and worked at different levels in their careers.

Today there are no limits, except that senior staff do not allow personal attacks and inconsiderate comments. Each member of the team knows they have the same rights and privileges at the meeting. Each expects the others to discuss each item in a fair and unbiased manner that will allow the team to make the best decision possible. They do not vote on items, although sometimes they talk about each person having one vote. They primarily do this to emphasize the fact that each of them has the same responsibility when it comes to evaluating proposals and the same responsibility for supporting a group decision. Their goal and commitment is to conduct discussions, as heated and passionate as they need to be, and then walk out of the room supporting the team's consensus and the mission of the hospital.

Those Tuesday morning breakfast club meetings were instrumental in the development of a servant leadership style at Bradley Memorial Hospital. The meetings also served as a microstudy of strategies that would foster the development of a hospitalwide management team. As time wore on, other collective meetings were scheduled, not always with the full team but frequently as circumstances warranted. The many issues that had traditionally been passed to the administrator were handed back to the complaining party with directions to meet and consider alternatives and solutions, and report back to "the management team" on Tuesday morning. Everything that affected the operation of the hospital was sent to that Tuesday morning meeting. It became so automatic that staff began to finish a sentence by saying, "I know, bring it to the team on Tuesday."

So senior staff collectively met for specific reasons and not always or solely for the purpose of solving day-to-day problems or for presetting next month or next year's management plan.

THE BENEFITS OF THE TUESDAY MORNING MEETINGS

Benefits of the consensus-building team sessions were these:

- Exposure.
- Consistency.
- Communication.
- Socialization.
- Group interaction.
- Development of self-confidence and elimination of the fear of failure.

There were other benefits, but these were the necessary elements for team building, developing relationships, and creating the servant leadership among the senior staff. In addition, there were individual meetings. It has been our experience that most hospital CEOs hold collective meetings but only practice making decisions during individual meetings. It is not difficult to see the negative implications of this double standard. And if not watched carefully, the individual meetings soon sabotage the collective meetings and destroy the integrity of the team.

ELIMINATING EMPLOYEE FEAR

So how did Whitlock structure individual meetings the first year of his administration?

> Very carefully. You see, some people were beating the door down to see me privately, while others avoided me in the hallway. Why? I would ask myself. The answer was—*fear*! You should recall that I had been exposed to all of these individuals for at least two years and most for three-and-a-half before becoming CEO. You would

think this to be a plus for them. How many staff members have three years to evaluate an individual who suddenly becomes the "Boss." If I had only just arrived, I could have understood their fear. In my mind I was no different than before I got the job. Why were they so afraid of me?

Eliminating this fear was a high priority for Whitlock. Although he wanted the team to feel comfortable making decisions without his input and to increase their confidence, he realized this could pose great hazards in certain circumstances. So they agreed the following rule of thumb would be applied. When an individual was placed in the position of making a major decision, by their definition of *major* (what was their comfort level in making the decision), they would ask themselves one question, "What's going to happen if I don't do anything right now?" The emphasis was placed on "right now." This was the philosophy on which Whitlock based his individual meetings. It began to give credit to the team in the eyes of the employees and it began to give credit and self-confidence to individuals on the management team. Fear was beginning to fade.

Here's a summary of Whitlock's steps during his first six to nine months on the job as CEO that would set the foundation for successful customer service later on:

1. Identification of the management team; who the players would be.
2. The mechanism by which they would communicate. What meetings they would have, and when they would have them; how they would be conducted.
3. The development of an annual management plan and a financial budget.
4. The coordinated efforts to continue the strategic plan that had been to a superficial level developed in 1989–90 and was now ready to be incorporated into the annual budget and management plan. It

now needed to be expanded to a site facility and a financial feasibility level.

5. A change in the relationship with the members of the board and the reporting of the management team at the regular board meeting. It also involved development of a unique relationship with department heads and supervisors to support and endorse the work that lay ahead for the long range plan.

At this point in the management development process, there was never any consideration as to how care would be delivered. There was never any consideration realistically of cultural change or philosophically changing how things were done. The evolution was just a matter of taking positions and letting team members learn more about each other. That took six to nine months to accomplish, but by the end of that period, every person on that senior team knew what Whitlock's style was; what his management philosophy was; and that it was probably credible.

DEVELOPING RELATIONSHIP WITH THE COMMUNITY

It was now time for Whitlock to begin developing a second relationship. That was the relationship with their community and with their county commissioners. In late 1989, the concept of a foundation became much more interesting to the board of trustees than it had ever been before. In late 1990, Jim began to pursue a formal foundation effort. Between July 1990 and the spring of 1991, formal efforts to create a foundation began to take place and ultimately an executive director, initially hired in a consulting capacity, was brought on board and made a permanent member of the management team.

By the end of the first year, a group of fairly comprehensive community representatives had been selected to help with the foundation and the board's enthusiasm over-flowed to the foundation's enthusiasm, and this group began to grow. This was an extremely important part of the customer service program. By early 1991, the foundation was beginning to grow, the strategic plan and its affiliated plans of financial feasibility and space planning were in place, architects and engineers had been selected, and team members were prepared to go to the county commission to begin this process.

At the end of several months, a collective meeting of all the county commissioners, the county executive, the local press, Whitlock's management team, his board members, and others launched what would be ultimately a $34-million major renovation and building plan for the hospital. Shortly thereafter, the county commission approved the largest bond issue in the history of the county at $6.7 million for the first phase of their project.

By early 1991, a third relationship began. Bradley leaders began talking about *guest services,* a new customer service culture, and how it could be achieved. Members of Whitlock's board, and specifically their board chairman, were motivated by the concept of guest services and had even expressed interest in having a mystery patient come to the hospital to evaluate the quality of their service and report to the management where the facility might improve. "He encouraged us to locate people who might do this. Quite honestly, that was difficult to do, but over a period of four to six months we were able to locate that individual; as you know this mystery patient was Dave Gorden," Jim told us.

The senior staff also began to talk about how much progress they, as a management team, had made in their relationship. They began to openly talk about the credibility of their relationship, the strength of working together, the trust they had developed, and all the important things that came along with this long-range strategic plan and the meetings associated with it. The weekly Tuesday sessions had been the medium within which they could work to develop this trust and this credibility. But their concern now was, how do they get this to the department head level? It was at this point Whitlock realized the issue was not how they *should* do it, but what was *keeping them* from doing it.

"BURYING ADMINISTRATION"

It occurred to Whitlock one day that the problem was *administration.*

> No matter where I went throughout the facility, it was not difficult to learn that "We can't do that because *administration* won't approve it," or "If we do this, *administration* may not like it" or "*Administration* doesn't allow this or they won't approve that or we can't do this, we can't do that because of *administration*," and it became apparent to me that we needed to get rid of *administration*.

Whitlock needed to effectively "bury administration." The next day he talked with Dewayne Belew about his crazy idea of "burying administration." Whitlock said, "Why don't you guys get together and think of a good way we could bury administration and make our point that we don't want administration to be a barrier any longer to our success?" Dewayne and Dan Gilbert, assistant administrator, came back to Whitlock with an idea that is probably not unique, but it was certainly a turning point in their relationship with those department heads and supervisors who worked with senior management. They decided they would videotape a funeral and bury administration in the process and that they would allow Whitlock the privilege of explaining to everyone why they had to bury administration as it now existed.

In order to present this "funeral," they had the first management retreat/educational conference of the hospital. Approximately 40 employees were invited to attend that first management retreat, and the attendees had absolutely no idea why they were being invited out of town for three days by senior management. When they arrived in Gatlinburg in 1991 and sat down to attend the opening presentation, they were greeted by a large-screen television set. On that the screen suddenly appeared an image of a graveyard with the administrator Jim Whitlock and funeral music being played in the background while the CEO walked through the graveyard.

As he stopped at an appropriate grave marker, Whitlock began to explain to the department heads and managers that the administrator could not join them today because he had to stay behind and conduct a funeral process that should not be perceived as sad, but rather be celebrated as a wake in the changing healthcare environment. He began to explain the need for change, the need for the redesign of the way staff deliver healthcare, and a change in the attitudes they have among those with whom they work. At the end of this presentation, the entire senior management team (eight of them) marched from behind a screen dressed in football uniforms and other appropriate garb and proceeded to pantomime a prerecorded rap demonstrating their various roles and responsibilities as senior management and projecting the need for team work, how they work together, and what they're going to do.

Basically they satirized themselves while making a point. Whitlock described it:

> We brought ourselves down to a level of humanness that this group of department heads had never experienced. At the termination of our presentation each one of us reached into a basket located at the front and we sailed tiny footballs labeled as the Bradley Memorial Management Team and we solicited their support in the development and growth of that team. To suggest that this was an ice breaker would be a significant understatement! For the remaining two days, they concentrated on the importance of team work and team building and

working together and it began an avalanche of opportunities among this group of people that has never slowed.

Lynn Dunlap, assistant administrator of nursing, remembers that management retreat as the turning point for the hospital:

> I believe the rapid changes started with that management retreat in 1991. At that meeting the administrative team decided that we wanted to be the preferred employer for healthcare in our region and we wanted to be the regional medical center! That's when we started to work toward the goal of employee buy-in. We worked on benefits and salaries. We started working with managers to develop their talents. We started involving employees in decision making. TQM began to be in vogue and we started developing our own version of TQM. TQM matched our management philosophy.

Craig Taylor, associate administrator and CFO, joined Bradley just as the new culture evolved in 1990:

> When I arrived in 1990, I found a culture that I perceived to be in transition. The most obvious to me was the change from a "not-for-profit" hospital to a hospital that strove to increase its profitability without sacrificing its mission. In order to achieve our profitability goals, we had to bring our employees into a new management philosophy that allowed participation in decision making. We began to accomplish this change gradually, but it began with our first management retreat when we buried administration.

Staff were truly becoming a family at Bradley Memorial Hospital. Barriers that created the fears and affected the creativity that reduced the productivity were slowly melting away along with the exterior facades that were so human to each of their personalities. They also began to expose this administrative staff to the new concepts of management being tossed about in the industry, specifically TQM/CQI, and the team-building concept itself. These strategies created a forum around which the staff could continue to develop this team-building attitude, this cultural relationship with the employees of the hospital, at least at the administrative staff level.

THE SAGA OF THE MYSTERY PATIENT

At about this time, the mystery patient paid a visit and a format was established for Customer Service Excellence through the Guest Excellence Task Force. The Guest Excellence Task Force provided an opportunity to develop some programs that would also satisfy the management goal of trying to promote this culture more deeply into the organization. Bradley's managers had spent the remainder of 1991 and all of 1992 concentrating on the administrative staff and supervisors at the department head levels, getting the team-building concept more or less adopted. They felt comfortable this was on its way. The team wanted to look at ways to further penetrate the organization with this culture.

The employee reorientation process gave Bradley's leaders an opportunity to bring all of the employees to a common point and discuss with them the mission of the hospital, pointing out the goals and objectives of the hospital. Managers also began to meet with selected employees, not at any supervisory level but just employees at a level of care giving and invite them to lunch with the administrator. They covered this on all three shifts throughout 1993 and early 1994. This was an effective way of using the grapevine to communicate the philosophies of not only the hospital but also the administrator, and this move gained attention and perhaps established some credibility in their relationship as a management team.

The task force came up with a concept used by staff trainers at Walt Disney World for employees, and from that picked up on the possibility of developing Bradley University, which would serve as a vehicle by which leaders would not only teach management skills but also communicate their vision of a serving culture and their team-building philosophy. "You may recall that my philosophy about management is that a manager has one responsibility and that is to identify what people do well and to give them an opportunity to do it," Whitlock explained. Bradley University offered the opportunity to take employees at the care-giving level, expose them to opportunities of promotion, opportunities of transition that would be more suited to their personalities, and ones more suited to their personal development needs. Although it's early in the implementation of Bradley University to confirm outcomes, there is marked enthusiasm among those who have completed the courses.

As it turned out, 1993 was a year of transition with employees as well as administrative staff. "I felt a much stronger relationship for the department heads. Our budgeting processes were much smoother. Our projections on budgeting were very accurate. We continued to reserve cash. We did an excellent job with our financial indicators. We were gaining strength with our board, our community, our foundation; and there were numerous celebrations with all of these groups," Whitlock explained.

Philosophically, staff were shedding the management-by-objectives (MBO) cloak. They were emphasizing the TQM task force concepts. They were training facilitators, talking about Bradley University, working into the Guest Excellence relationship, and reorienting employees to these concepts. All of 1993 was designed to bring the employees in the relative departments up to speed with administrative management, the department heads, and senior supervisors. By 1993, the one-day brainstorming session that began as the management team retreat had moved to a two-day session. This made the opportunity to build their team even stronger.

TRANSFORMING THE EMERGENCY ROOM INTO A "SUPER DEPARTMENT"

In 1994, Bradley's leaders began to talk seriously about the reengineering concepts of the hospital. Although managers really didn't know what reengineering was, they began to use terms like *Super Department;* began to look for people within the administrative management team who could help design and develop relationships to support a Super Department. Their educational efforts were directed toward rethinking their management plan, getting away from MBO and even possibly TQM/CQI concepts, and modifying them or customizing them a bit more (but most assuredly in budgeting).

As 1994 came to a close, the renovation of the emergency department (ED) was high priority. This department had demonstrated the opportunity for team building and working together. They were forced to remodel 10,000 square feet of the second busiest emergency center in the southeast United States. Task forces that had been trained to function and operate under the previous TQM systems pulled it off without a hitch. As 1995 began, leaders continued to see the benefit of their early efforts developing their management team. Whitlock summed it up:

> We also see some problems that we are having to address as we become more and more accustomed to working in this environment with each other and we become more used to each other. We begin to take each other more for granted and we also begin to second guess each other in terms of what we do and what we don't do. These are things we've had to transition to as well.

So now, after five years of learning how to work together, Bradley's leaders now emphasize how they *keep* working together and how they *remain* supportive team members as well as friends in this whole relationship.

Craig Taylor, associate administrator, looks at it this way: "The key to this change in culture basically boils down to relationships. If you can develop an honest, trusting, mutually beneficial relationship with your staff, then there is nothing your organization can't accomplish. The key to our success has been relationships."

We told Jim Whitlock we were going to try to explain how his servant leadership style laid the groundwork for successful customer relations at Bradley. We told him we were going to try to "put a box around" the concept so the readers of this book could determine how to emulate what worked so well at this hospital. His response was,

> You have asked me on more than one occasion what the cookie cutter concept is that has created the environment you experienced during your visit, which has resulted in the successes we have enjoyed at Bradley Memorial Hospital over the past five years. My response to you has been consistently *relationships*. I understand this is not what people want to read in a book. It's really too simple. It's also at the same time too complex to be a good answer, but it must begin there. As we talk about penetrating culture, what we're really talking about doing is developing relationships so that they can in effect change the culture. Unfortunately, the need to transition and to change culture takes a great deal of time, and providers in healthcare don't have a great deal of time.

10
CHAPTER

Focus on Customer Service

About the same time Bradley Memorial Hospital was changing the management culture and beginning to empower the employees in a variety of ways, their focus also zeroed in on customer service. It was like two major culture conversions going on at the same time: internally with employees and externally with healthcare customers. Actually, the nudge toward the customer service focus came from the hospital board chairman, Sam Bettis. While driving home together from a meeting in early 1991, Bettis suggested to Jim Whitlock that the hospital look into finding someone to pose as a patient and investigate the facility's customer service first hand. Whitlock, in turn, turned the project of finding someone who did such investigations over to Lynn Dunlap, assistant administrator and director of nursing. She found that someone in Dave Gorden, a healthcare consultant specializing in customer service.

In June 1991 a patient was routinely admitted to the hospital. As far as everyone at the hospital was concerned, his admission was no different from any of the thousands made throughout the years. However, this patient was actually a hired professional who had been a mystery patient in some 35 hospitals (a total now exceeding 50) throughout the United States for more than 11 years. "It was very difficult to keep this a secret, but we knew the entire purpose of his hospital stay would be defeated if too many people knew," said Dunlap. The imposter's mission at Bradley was to evaluate every aspect of the hospital from finding the correct place to park, to discharge arrangements, and discussion of his final bill. The "sting" operation would conclude on the Tuesday following his weekend stay with the patient's true identity revealed and a full report presented by the mystery patient Dave Gorden to all hospital department heads and managers at an off-site retreat. "My only concern was that I did not want our staff or physicians to think we were merely trying to catch things being done wrong," Dunlap said. "That was not our objective. Our objective was to lay the groundwork for changing the hospital's culture."

While at the hospital, the mystery patient encountered the same types of experiences that happen every day in hospitals everywhere. To document his stay, Gorden took copious notes when staff members were not present. Although he found isolated areas in need of improvement, he also discovered exceptional examples of customer service. "We found some departments that were doing a superb job," Dunlap stated. "At the same time, we discovered some areas where there were opportunities for changing our systems and providing additional training for our employee."

Gorden recalled what led up to the hospital stay and his three-day inpatient experience:

> I always tell a hospital administrator I'm not going to tell you what you want to hear, I'm going to tell you what you need to know. Jim was very open to that. When I was discharged three days later, as is my practice, the CEO and I go out to lunch somewhere and talk about the

experience. I asked Jim, "How do you want me to handle it at the department head meeting tomorrow?" He said, "I want you to handle it the way it happened. I want them to hear it and I want you to share it."

Gorden presented his findings in a positive, upbeat manner to the senior staff and department heads at a management retreat, never skirting the negative experiences but discussing them as *systems* problems, not *individual* shortcomings. At the conclusion of the meeting, the senior staff and all department heads agreed that the next step should be creating a culture where all employees, volunteers, and physicians were treated like "guests." The theory behind this was if the staff and volunteers were well treated and recognized for their efforts, patients would be the ultimate beneficiary, because the treatment would be repeated. It set the foundation for what would follow—improved employee relationships and improved customer service.

DEVELOPMENT OF THE GUEST EXCELLENCE TASK FORCE

Based on the consultant's report and information gained at the retreat, the hospital put together a special group of employees they called the Guest Excellence Task Force. Department heads and supervisors who wanted to volunteer for the Task Force were asked to submit a one-page letter stating why they wanted to be a member. From the letters submitted, 10 people from various departments were chosen. Jim Whitlock was not a member of the task force, which turned out to be a good decision.

Dave Gorden explained Whitlock's nonrole on the task force:

> Jim really wanted to be on this task force. But let me qualify this—there was nothing that ever went on—that a conclusion was reached that Jim does not know about. When we had discussions and a little dynamic tension, I said the group recommends that, or we'd like to do such

and such. We certainly never excluded him, and he did get a report on every meeting. However, it would hamper the procedure if the administrator were in the meeting. Jim trusted us, but he's a hands-on kind of guy—he really wanted to be there.

At the task force's first meeting, a consensus was reached that internal guests—employees, volunteers, and physicians—initially would be the primary focus of all task force work. This was a key decision and in keeping with the culture change going on with the employees. "If we do not treat each other with respect and show courtesy toward one another, how can we expect to change the hospital's culture? By focusing on our internal guests, we would make dramatic changes in the way we serve our patients. You can still feel how things are improving," Dunlap explained.

During the course of the first year, the task force implemented four Guest Excellence focused projects:

• In the first month, task force members conducted the enormous task of reorientation sessions for 1,159 hospital employees and volunteers. During the three-hour sessions, participants were informed about the hospital's mission, the new 12-point Guest Excellence creed, and asked to complete a 24-question fun-but-educational quiz about the hospital.

Near the end of each session, each participant was presented with a new hospital name badge that featured the employee's or volunteer's face, their full name, title, and their first name in print large enough to be seen from 20 feet away. "Putting our names out there for everyone to see does two things. First, anyone we encounter can quickly identify us. Second, when you realize that everyone knows who you are there is incentive to do the best you can," Dunlap explained.

Reorientation turned out not to be a one-time event. The task force regularly evaluates the program's content so when presented to new employees and volunteers each month, the information is current and consistent. Additionally, a hospitalwide reorientation for all employees and volunteers was conducted again by the former mystery patient.

Prior to concluding each session, each employee was asked to sign a large sign that stated in bold letters, "I Am Committed to Guest Excellence at Bradley Memorial Hospital." Following the classroom reorientation, each group was taken on a one-hour tour of the hospital, with special emphasis placed on areas of new technology and departments not usually seen.

• To immediately recognize true Guest Excellence, Applause-A-Grams were produced. It was determined that this award could be passed to anyone who was deemed worthy of recognition. The second program, called Bunny Bucks, recognized Guest Excellence and included a financial reward. Anyone who received Bunny Bucks (similar to Disney Dollars and featuring the hospital's mascot, Brad Lee Bunny) could cash them in for a free meal in the hospital cafeteria or a discount in the hospital giftshop. Catchers were identified on each shift throughout the hospital. These were the individuals who observed and rewarded employees they caught in the act of some aspect of favorable customer service. Additionally, all persons who were caught each month were eligible for a cash award. At the end of the year, the names of all "caught" persons were placed in a drawing to receive a vacation of their choice.

• The hospital began hosting grassroots meetings between the hospital administrator and 12 employees randomly chosen from different departments.

IMMEDIATE IMPROVEMENT IN GUEST EXCELLENCE

Was Bradley's work over the first year successful or worth the workhours spent brainstorming, developing, fine tuning, implementing, and monitoring this Guest Excellence process? Morale was up (based on a SESCO employee opinion survey). Patient complaints were down. The hospital had its best financial year since it opened in 1952. The facility completed the largest construction project in the hospital's history. More new physicians joined the hospital staff in 1991–92. By many standards, the answer was an astounding yes.

Lynn Dunlap explained to us that the focus on improved customer service was triggered by the mystery patient experience:

> Part of all this activity was the mystery patient experience. I was fortunate to find someone with a positive attitude, motivational speaking skills, and the ability to help us develop customer service programs to sell our philosophy. If the mystery patient experience had been presented in a negative fashion or the "I've got you attitude," the outcome would have set us back five years.

However, the customer service programs are just a small piece of it. Programs are just a way of internal marketing. Internal marketing is very important but pales in comparison to living the philosophy. *Living* the philosophy is the key. Employees are valued and are considered to be team members. How can that not help but spill over to customers? Most people are in the healthcare field because they really want to help people. Bradley has proven that if you create the environment for employees to do that, the customer service naturally follows.

In 1994, the Guest Relations Task Force unveiled Bradley University. Bradley University is a comprehensive management training program—the only one of its kind at a healthcare organization as far as Bradley has been able to determine. The program offers managers and aspiring managers the opportunity for professional and personal growth and development. Dave Gorden recalled the birth of the idea for the Bradley University:

It was something that Jim Whitlock had seen as a need, and I think this is true everywhere in healthcare. What we tend to do in healthcare is we take good clinicians and technicians and promote them to management, but we don't *train* them to be management. And so, many times they fail. We do that in industry as well, but it's really rampant in healthcare. We take someone who was a good technician and we make him a manager. Now they no longer get to do the technical aspects, but they have to manage other people and get results with and through other people. They don't know how because we never trained them.

We asked Jim Whitlock at what point he realized who the hospital's customer is. Did he know that from the beginning?

You know something? And I said this to the president of HCA one time. HCA's mission statement way back when I started 11 years ago, was to have a fair return to the shareholder. That was it. I believe you do what this hospital does. They talk about quality of care, they talk about commitment to their team members, internally first, and then externally, they talk about guest excellence. Some organizations say, the way we're going to make a profit is we're going to cut your hours back, we're going to lay you off. Now go out there and take good care of our patients. It won't happen. The commitment has to be internally to employees first.

The bottom line is that Bradley understood that until staff take care of the internal customer, they can never take care of the external customer. And the commitment here is to the internal customer.

PUBLIC RELATIONS PRIMARY STRATEGIES

With the hospital's commitment to enhancing customer service within the organization, managers have allocated about 40 percent of the marketing and public relations budget to internal education, marketing, communications, and celebrations. Although they focused a great deal of effort to the development of their internal market, at the same time managers enhanced their efforts in the external market. The primary strategies they followed included improved media relations, paid advertising, and community outreach programs and education. All of these strategies had one objective: heightened awareness about the Bradley Memorial Hospital staff, facility improvements, state-of-the-art technology, role in the community as a "good" neighbor, and healthy growth of the medical staff.

The hospital positioned itself through a major marketing campaign as being the medical center that is "Miles Ahead. Minutes Away." In these four words Bradley attempted to take advantage of its centralized location in the market (minutes away). Through Miles Ahead the staff attempted to communicate the fact that their people are advanced in training and compassion and their facility and technology are state-of-the-art. This campaign has served as the basis for all of Bradley's advertising since 1992. For the campaign the marketing people created a musical identity that says a great deal about Bradley. The tune is up-tempo with instrumentals and vocals:

> Something is happening,
> Medicine's moving at a rapid pace.
> Technology's changing.
> A better Bradley is built today.
> Bradley Memorial Hospital. Miles Ahead. Minutes Away.
> Caring for your family.
> Bradley Memorial,
> Miles Ahead. Minutes Away.

By focusing on customer service in a variety of ways and by having two "customers"—the employee and the patient—Bradley certainly seems miles ahead of most providers in excelling in customer relations.

GUEST EXCELLENCE CREED AT BRADLEY MEMORIAL

1. I am a team player. As a member of the team, I provide with care and concern the professional service that my guests deserve.

   Guest Excellence takes the effort of all team members at Bradley Memorial Hospital. You are a very important player on this team. No matter what your job title may be, it takes all of us, working together, every day, in every way, to provide the very best service.

2. I speak to my guests with my voice and my eyes. I handle complaints without becoming defensive.

   Every complaint is an opportunity. It means that something is not just as it should be and we have a chance to make it right. A pleasant tone of voice goes a long way in helping our guests know that we really do care.

3. I smile at my guests to show that I welcome them and to help put them at ease.

   A friendly smile lets everyone know that we want him/her to feel good. It also tells others that we are happy to be there to help them. (By the way, you burn up 10 calories every time you smile.)

4. I listen to my guests with my ears, my eyes—in fact with all of my body, except my voice. Even if it's "Not my job," I will *help* or *find someone who can.*

   Our guests don't always tell us exactly what is bothering them; we should always look at them when they are speaking to us. We must always do whatever it takes to make our guests happy.

5. I introduce myself to my guests and explain what I am doing and why, to reduce anxiety.

   People are often afraid of what they don't understand. By telling a guest who you are and what

   (Continued)

you are going to do, it helps them know that you are a concerned professional.

6. I am always considerate of the feelings of my guests, and I don't talk about my guests or their case in public places. I do everything in my power to respect their dignity.

    A guest who overhears part of a conversation may think that you are talking about them or someone in their family. We always want everyone to know that we respect his/her privacy.

7. I am courteous to my guests by allowing them to go first through doors and into elevators and by keeping the halls as quiet as possible.

    The Golden Rule really does work; "we should always do unto others as we would have them do unto us."

8. I am alert to give service, directions, and assistance. I anticipate the needs of my guests.

    If we see people who look like they need help, let's smile at them and offer to assist them. Remember, our hospital is very large and it is often difficult to find certain areas.

9. I always call guests by name, because they deserve my personal attention.

    A person's name is the sweetest, most important sound he/she hears. Let's call our fellow team members by name whenever possible. Look at their ID badge and use their name; you will be surprised at how good we can make each other feel.

10. I project a caring attitude.

    We are in the healthcare profession because we sincerely care about other people. We must always do everything we can to let people know we care. "People do not care how much you know, until they know how much you care."

(Concluded)

11. I look the part by dressing professionally in a manner appropriate to my position.

    We must demonstrate the pride that we feel for our hospital and the pride that we take in ourselves with the image that we project. Our outside appearance projects the image of our team.

12. I always treat my guests with care, imagining that I am on the receiving end. I will care for my guests as though they were my family or friends.

    Once again, the Golden Rule applies. Always ask yourself, if this were my mother or father, brother or sister, what would I do? That goes for all of our guests, including our fellow team members.

SPECIFIC CUSTOMER SERVICE ACTIONS AND TIME FRAMES

Before the Mystery Patient

1985: Get Nice classes: A video was shown about a patient named Joe Green. A facilitator led a discussion about what a difference staff could have made in his hospital stay. Was not a big hit with the employees. Too superficial.

1987: Get Nice classes held for the emergency department. Outside facilitator attempted to aid staff in dealing with upset customers, but the employee evaluations of the program were generally stated: "You don't understand what we are dealing with."

1990: Emergency department held group therapy sessions with an outside facilitator to deal with problems related to ER guest relations and supervisor relations on a feeling level. These were termed somewhat successful in that at least the staff did feel "heard."

After the Mystery Patient

March 1991:	Management retreat: First formal efforts at team building and making managers feel special.
June 1991:	Mystery patient entered hospital. Retreat held with department managers to discuss findings.
July 1991:	Requested letters from managers interested in Guest Excellence Task Force.
August 1991 through February 1992:	Task force developed guest excellence creed and reorientation program.
March 1992:	Task force worked on catcher program.
April 1992:	Management retreat, continued to focus on team building, cooperation, and front-line involvement. Reinforced that Guest Excellence must begin with each other and it will naturally flow to external customers.
May 1992:	Implemented catcher program.
June 1992:	Visited by another hospital to review Bradley's rapid progress.
August 1992:	Implemented grassroots meetings.
September 1992 to March 1993:	Task force changed the catcher program. Balloon bouquets were the reward for getting caught beginning in July.

July 1993:   Reorientation in July to keep the momentum up.

The task force began developing Bradley University in order to give managers the tools to enable them to be even better managers.

September 1993:   New catchers oriented and in place. New Bunny Bucks program in place by July 1994.

April 1994:   Bradley University concept presented to department heads at Educational Conference.

August 1994:   Developed float design for ER parade.

October 1994:   Bradley University began classes.

March 1995:   Objectives for guest relations outlined for upcoming year.

May 1995:   Action plan developed for objectives.

11

CHAPTER

Sanction Employees to Serve—Mind, Body, and Soul

The beauty of the success of customer service at Bradley Memorial Hospital is the way it is "practiced" by employees throughout the organization. During our week-long visit at the hospital, we interviewed all the senior management staff, most of the department heads, some supervisors, several board members, and many nonmanagement employees. We walked the halls, sat in the waiting rooms, ate in the cafeteria, and lingered in the lobby. What we found was a genuine fixation about patient satisfaction and how important it was in employees' roles.

They live it mind, body, and soul.

Our conclusion is that truly successful customer service can be accomplished when employees feel good about themselves and their jobs *first*. Attempts to sandwich customer service around disgruntled, uninspired, unenthusiastic employees will likely fall apart. Employees will see the sandwich approach as another flavor-of-the-month or view customer service as another "program" hospital administration is pushing on the employees. They say, "Take care of me first and I'll take good care of the patient and all aspects of customer service for you. I'll do it because I want to, not because you want me to." What employees universally want from their employer and senior management is a chance to have input into the decision-making process, and acknowledgment of their contribution; in short, to be needed, heard, and cared about. They want to be listened to and have action taken on their concerns.

When that's accomplished, employees fall all over themselves to provide excellent customer service—particularly if the organization shines its headlights on customer service and repeats over and over how important it is and the reasons why. The employee actually becomes *sanctioned* to or empowered (there's that overused word again) to serve the patient in a fashion that goes far beyond the norm. Customer service becomes something that comes naturally. It is a natural extension of their thought process, and their actions play out their beliefs.

These conclusions really don't sound complicated. Achieving customer service goals does take time, though. It is definitely not a quick-fix approach. It is not complicated; however, it's not practiced at most of the hospitals and clinics in which we worked as consultants. This approach may not be described as the "normal" path most providers take to improve customer service, but it certainly is effective. More providers should concentrate on empowering or sanctioning employees to exercise care and concern for their customers on their own terms so employees develop an ownership in the process. It is the truest form of customer service.

HOW GOOD CUSTOMER SERVICE PERMEATES THE ENTIRE HOSPITAL

In preceding chapters we have spelled out the process that led to excellent customer service at Bradley—how it started with a management cultural conversion coupled with a concentrated focus on customer service. But the final piece of the puzzle is how the practice of good customer service permeates through the employees in the organization. The many interviews we had with department heads, supervisors, and employees reflect the notion that good customer service takes place at all levels. We sensed employees felt empowered to do what had to be done. We have chosen a few representative interviews that best reflected the employees' responses.

Nursing Manager

Edna Shepherd, RN, nursing supervisor of 4N at Bradley, told us, "That was one of the things when we first started: that they were talking about empowering the managers, that we had to be educated to begin to realize that this really is our niche; that we are really responsible, really are in charge, really have some authority, and really have a voice." A nursing veteran, Shepherd told us she slowly began to change the way she managed. "I think our staff had to see it from us . . . it changed the way I manage . . . I mean, literally. Because I have a strong personality, I'm an authoritarian, and I thought, do I really want to be the kind of person who treats my staff that way?"

We asked Edna Shepherd to tell us about the transition for her as a manager and her approach toward her employees and theirs to the patients and their families. What promoted the transition, and how did it change her management style? She replied, "I think part of it was the change of philosophy from upper management. There was a whole change of philosophy. Suddenly they are sharing things with us that they had never shared before. They were looking at me as capable of doing more than I had ever done before . . . they were looking at me differently . . . so I began to look at myself differently."

Shepherd thought the feedback from the patient surveys also had an impact on the employees' focus on patient satisfaction. "Another thing that helped us perceive was the patient survey . . . when they started to put out the patient survey and we started to get back what people were really saying about us. It was a little startling, but it had a big impact on me. All of a sudden I'm looking at this differently . . . because you can hear rumblings and my staff saying, 'They just drove us crazy the whole time they were here.' Now we were hearing it for the first time from our patient's perspective or their family's perspective," she explained.

Shepherd described her feelings about what the patients were saying:

> In the beginning it was hard for me because I was still in this codependent management relationship style that I was responsible for everybody, and it made me feel as if I was a really poor manager because my staff wasn't "at par," they weren't doing what they should do. In the beginning it was mind-boggling for me. But, as I really got to look at it—it's really funny because I teach overcoming codependency classes—I had never placed codependency in the workplace. All of a sudden I'm saying to myself, "You made a lot of changes in your home or whatever, but you're as codependent in the workplace as anything I've ever seen."

We inquired how she perceived that she was codependent in this situation. "Because I took on total responsibility for the actions of my staff. As long as I took on total responsibility nobody else could grow. I couldn't grow as the middle-manager as long as upper-management had total responsibility. People can't grow unless you take down some walls. You have to be able to make mistakes, you have to be able to learn, and I've made some. I've made some good ones. But I'm still here." As her management style changed, the defensive barriers toward patient criticism came down. Shepherd and her staff began to look at patient complaints in a different light:

I think our staff meetings changed. We started to talk about the comments in the patient surveys and going over them. Then we would talk about situations and we began to really look at what we can do to improve. We actually started to look at it in a different way, trying not to be so defensive. You can never see your own mistakes in an accurate light as long as you're defensive.

We asked Shepherd how she and her employees conquered defensiveness and resistance to change:

In the beginning I think my staff thought I was kind of cruel, because what I would do is play devil's advocate. For instance, if they started griping about patient complaints, I'd say, "Yes, but look at it from their side." I think it was a matter of education. In some cases we actually sent nurses to the pharmacy to visit for three or four hours. They watched them work and saw what they had to do. They had to cross over those lines so they could better understand each other. We sent some nurses to admitting, watching the process, watching what happens there. Those were some of the things that were done. I really think it was like a gradual education-type thing.

Another (nonmanagement) nursing employee told us, "When all the changes in guest excellence were going on, I was still a staff person at that time and it was no big flash for me. I remember when the emphasis on Guest Relations first came out it was kind of a joke—we had the first 'revival' meeting. As things kept on, there was a gradual change. We stopped looking at the patients as causing us problems."

Nursing Staff

One of the more direct, open discussions we had was with Gary Thomas, a recovery room RN. A large, well-built man with a dark beard speckled with gray, Thomas told us he had been with the hospital a long time and had seen the change in culture and attitudes toward fellow employees and patients. We asked him to discuss customer service and patient satisfaction from his point of view.

> I know if you treat people with respect and treat them how you would like to be treated it works a lot better and you get things done. The families feel better and the patients feel better, but sometimes it's still hard for me to do this.
>
> If you are going to do this, you have to gain the patients' confidence, you have to gain their trust. You have to be nice. I think sometimes you can even fake it. If you have to do that, fine. It gets to be a habit and gets to be where you are sincere. I'm not a cheerleader, but I have reached the stage if I decide to stay in nursing, I'm going to have to change.

We asked Thomas why he thought he had to change:

> To be able to exist and have a job and to even have a hospital we're going to have to change and that scares me . . . and that has to do with money, job security, and all of that. Now things are changing to where I might not get to work five days a week if our census is low. I've got to remember I've been told to be flexible, and as I get older I'm not that flexible. So I'm going to have to change. The big difference we've seen and learned is that through guest excellence we can get our work done a lot better if we just take families in on the front line, teach them what they need to know, try to settle their fears and deal with it from there. Patients are so much more aware of things they weren't two to five years ago. They expect a certain amount of things and a certain amount of information and help.

We wanted Thomas' thoughts about how the value of the employee was increased. The organizational culture at Bradley indicated that if the employees feel good about their jobs, feel that they have a lot more input in decision-making processes, and have bought into the culture as far down as senior management can take it, that employees will do the tasks that they sense are important, not only clinically but also in customer service. Thomas summarized it:

> It will work. It took us a while . . . this is so new, and nurses do not want to change. At first I thought it was a bunch of hooey and sometimes I still do, but I think it's one of those things you really believe in, even if we do have to fake it for a while until it starts working.

Thomas reflects the whole idea that if employees feel better about their jobs as employees in the front-line, customer service improves. He concluded: "I think it filters down . . . and you start to develop that feeling, an attitude toward your work and kind of the spiritual, emotional thing. You show it, other people sense it."

Medical Records and Laboratory Staff

As we tried to get the employees to describe their experiences during the culture conversion, we had an interesting exchange with Nancy Dees, medical records director, and Gail Ownby, cardiac cath labs.

Here are the highlights of that interview:

Q: If you were to compare the customer service that you had five or six years ago (10 is high, 1 is low), what would the score be then, and how would you score it today?

A: Probably a 4 and a 9.9.

Q: How do you go from a 4 to a 9.9? Can you tell me in a paragraph? Summarize it? What are the major ingredients?

A: I think Guest Excellence starts with an intelligent person who recognizes potential in employees.

Q: But how did it go from a 4 to a 9.9?

A: I think one of the things was establishing relationships. Walls came down.

Q: What does it have to do with guest relations, though? You're saying generally the difference is that administration is open, the walls came down. But what does that have to do with guest relations?

A: If all of us are happy, challenged, doing a good job . . . we are more capable of practicing good customer service. You can't do it in steps, you can't one–two–three it. You can't give, step one this will happen. Step two this is what happens.

Q: Did you feel differently? Did you, yourselves, others around you, your peers, feel differently toward the patient, in a sense?

A: Well, I think part of it is giving ownership to the employee. Remember, Guest Excellence is everyone's responsibility. Suddenly, we're allowed some freedom. You could speak your mind. We were given ownership. The first thing you do is give employees ownership of their lives. Once you give them ownership of their lives, leadership is easy. You set parameters, you set the deadlines, you tell them what has to be done, when, and how many days you've got to get it done, and give them ownership of it. Now this is the end product. However you get to that, once you're trained, is your choice.

Q: Help me with some confusion. Okay, you're saying what separates you from others is that there's a new management philosophy, and that's great. But I want you to help me understand how opening up—and this participative management where you were given freedom, and you were given input and you were not afraid to make mistakes because you didn't get your head chopped off—is really customer service. Help me see that.

> A: *I think that before, we tried to make things work*
> *more efficiently; we tried to take good care of our*
> *patients. I care for the patients the way I've*
> *always cared for them. That hasn't changed. But*
> *I wasn't given the freedom or the empowerment*
> *or autonomy to go ahead and do the* extra. *For*
> *example, a surgeon wasn't going to get this*
> *patient in on time, we had some scheduling*
> *problems going across the board, and maybe we*
> *could provide this family with breakfast in our*
> *cafeteria. You would think of these ideas, but you*
> *wouldn't say anything because years ago that*
> *would have been nipped in the bud, "No, we can't*
> *do that. That's unheard of!" Now, you say*
> *something about that and they do it. When you're*
> *full of fear, maybe we didn't serve these people as*
> *well as we should have, or, at least the nurses*
> *section; this is reality to them. If we can go ahead*
> *and do this, you're not stifled in your ideas on*
> *how you can better care for that patient.*

Nursing Supervisors

We asked many of the nonmanagement employees their impression of the cultural changes and what impact they thought CEO Jim Whitlock or his senior management team had on the transition. Responses that rather typified most of the replies were from Beverly Dunn and Dorothy Phillips, both nursing supervisors.

> Q: What do you sense in your position, and you've
> been here for a long time, what difference did the
> CEO Jim Whitlock make?
> A: *He had a different approach to the whole*
> *management system. I think his approach was a*
> *hit: He said it's okay to have fun; we've got*
> *business to do, but we can have fun doing it. He*

also stretched our paradigms to think. He told us we're not just this little entity. As a hospital, we have to reach out to the community. He's talked about that from almost day one. What you do or say when you leave here makes a difference. We want you to be visible in the community, because we've got people here that have a lot of expertise that can help in the community.

I think that Jim is a true leader because he was able to lead us toward knocking down those administration walls that existed for so many years. He believed in that slow, patient approach, which I think helped us. I think employees have to see you, know you, and sense everything's okay before they start to trust you. I think he allowed us to have our own dreams and our own visions, even though he had his own. Somehow, we meshed those together. He didn't take away our self-worth while he was building what he called his new environment. We all had a part in the building process. He allowed us to be a part of that, and to feel a part of that. I see him as a leader because he's our administrator, but he's also our friend.

Q: You made an interesting comment earlier: It flows down hill; guest excellence has to flow downhill. What did you mean by that?

A: Well, no matter what I do as a nurse manager, if my staff or my patients see Lynn (my administrator of nursing) as being off-limits, untouchable, unapproachable, not touching, not friendly, whatever, it stops right there. If you have this same focus all the way down the organization it makes it stronger. If some part of that ladder is broken, then it weakens the whole ladder. So basically, it has to be strong to flow down.

Q: What does customer service mean to you? What
do you look for? What are the factors that make
up good guest excellence?

*A: For me, it goes beyond how my nurses, or my
nursing assistants, or my attendants treat the
patient and the family. It's how staff put them at
ease, make them feel comfortable, let them know
that we're here to serve them. That's what we do—
we serve—and we're going to use the word* serve
*in the element it should be. We're here to take care
of their needs. It goes beyond that. It's how they
treat each other as employees. Because if they are
not cohesive as a group, it's not going to be
reflected in your overall care for the patient.
That's the key for me. For me, patient satisfaction
is that family environment, where everyone has a
part and a role to play. It's not a role you're
playing, that's you. You become that person that
is patient satisfaction.*

*Even things as small as seeing a piece of paper
on the floor—before, I've seen people just walk on
by and it's no big deal. For the longest time, we
had a lot of cigarette butts on the front steps of
the hospital. It was so interesting to have our
staff complain that it just doesn't look right, it's
not a good image for us. Now, anyone and
everyone picks up those cigarette butts and paper
on the floors. It's also the little things that go
toward good customer service. For us, we began to
see everyone here receiving the treatment and the
care you would give to your family—your mom,
your dad, your brother, your sister. That's what
Guest Excellence is all about.*

*We've always had it ingrained in us to give
patients good quality care, but we didn't have
ingrained in us how important we were to the
hospital. When they came out with Guest*

Excellence, they presented it to the employees that
you're guests too. We want you to be happy,
because we want you to stay with us and be part
of our family. Everyone felt better . . .
immediately.

Q: In your minds, what are the most important
factors in customer service? What are the key
ingredients that would identify excellence in
patient relations?

A: *It's like providing satisfaction, a satisfied*
customer. You know when you get, we call them
warm fuzzies sometimes, when they come back,
they call you, they send you flowers, they send
letters to your employer telling you what a nice
unit the hospital has.

Q: What do you do, though, that creates this?

A: *Showing that you truly care about patients.*
You're not there just to do a job, to do the
procedures. You go that extra mile. You care
about them as people. Touch individual people.
Let them realize that we know that they have
needs and we want to help meet those needs.

Q: Let me ask you a few final questions. If
somebody said, "I want to develop a better
customer service program in my hospital," would
you tell them that one of the first things you've
got to do—I don't want to overuse this word—
empower or develop ownership, get your
employees to see all aspects of the job? As you
get employees to take ownership in all aspects,
and they feel good about what they're doing, all
the things you've talked about here, what it takes
to develop this ownership on the job, that one of
the things that spins off is their concern for all of
the things that make up good customer service.
Say that somebody came in and asked you, "If I

want to develop a customer service program,
where do I start?" Do they start with the
employees? Not the patient, not the customer?

A: *Yes, I think so. I think the emphasis is already
there in healthcare—of taking care of the patient.
I would say in most facilities, the place that they
would need to look into is taking care of their
employees. The natural follow-through is they're
going to take care of the patient.*

That's where customer service begins and it never
ends.

SUMMARY

It's difficult, if not impossible, to capture the process and
experiences that led to successful customer service at Bradley Memorial Hospital, to create some kind of script that
other providers could follow. Don't misunderstand, Bradley
is not perfect in all aspects of customer service. The facility
still has some warts, like every institution does. A few
employees still don't get it. Problems with patient complaints still crop up. But this hospital is far more advanced
than most of the nation's providers, based on our recent
research and our many years spent as employees and consultants in hospitals. We feel Bradley's success in developing improved patient relations is worth studying and
emulating.

First, based on Bradley's successful approach, customer
service should be considered a *state of mind*. Employees
should see it as a *mindset* so that providing good service
comes as naturally as possible. It should not be seen as a
program, policy, or some kind of be-nice-to-patients plati-
tude that is thrust upon the employees by senior management. The employees will see through those approaches and
chuckle at the idea behind your back. They laugh because
the emphasis on customer service doesn't make sense unless
the *employees feel cared for first*. Employees have to know

they come first in terms of concern, compassion, being listened to, communicated with, become part of decision making, and—most of all—trusted.

The ostentatious walls of arrogance that administration often builds around itself must come down to develop this new culture. This haughty behavior manifests disdain by the employees and creates an environment of superficiality and disgust. It creates a lack of trust between the employees and administration and bottles up the serving, sharing attitude so necessary in successful patient relations. Outstanding service in an organization starts with servant leadership at the top.

Chuck Lauer, publisher of *Modern Healthcare*, spelled out his thoughts on good leadership in one of his publisher's letters:

> It all starts with humility. By that I mean not taking yourself too seriously. Too many executives think their organizations would fall apart were it not for their talent and dedication. They don't want to share power because they're too insecure about their own abilities. Even more important is the desire to treat your colleagues and customers with a gentleness that inspires confidence and loyalty. For some people that's hard to do because they feel vulnerable when they show their emotions. It's all very easy, but it requires the leader to be with his people, not in some office on the top floor where there's no noise and no laughter and where everyone is afraid to say anything for fear of being criticized or ridiculed. Good leaders know where their people are and what they need because they're good listeners.[1]

Developing an attitude of serving others has to run downhill. The example must be set by the CEO and the entire senior staff, particularly the director of nursing and vice-presidents of all the ancillary departments. Employees

---

1. Charles Lauer, publisher's letter, *Modern Healthcare,* November 1993.

will need to see this servant attitude consistently played out before they will be receptive to serving patients and their families in the manner that could be identified as excellent service. Employees have to "feel" it first. Great customer service starts with an organizational culture that stresses relationships and cultivates trust among all levels of employees, from the CEO through the executive staff, department heads, managers, supervisors, and each employee. The CEO has to initiate this process of nurturing relationships and service to one another throughout the organization, consistently and continuously.

The CEO also has to paint the vision for the future of the organization for the employees and breathe the passion of organizational pride into their very souls. Pride in the place you work is important. It is a key link in creating employee desire to excel at customer service. Once the culture of the organization has impacted the employees to the point where they feel like "guests" in their own organization—where they feel good about their organization, their contributions and their relationship with each other—then they will be receptive to excelling in customer service. This would be the time to throw in specific customer service activities, such as task forces, training, and developing specific ideas for improving patient relations. In fact, in this environment employees themselves will take patient relations to a level no other process could properly achieve. Employees will see themselves as a family and patients as guests in their "house." And a family treats guests as special while they are visiting in their "house." The more the internal "guests" feel the warmth, caring, sincere relationships with one another and administration, the more they will be able to give of themselves to the patients.

It's pretty much as simple as that. But as Jim Whitlock stated, that's not what readers want to read. But that's where it starts—building relationships with employees—and ends in developing relationships with patients who will

be coming back again and again. Following is our attempt
at fitting Bradley's experiences to a step-by-step process
that may enable others to mirror the "process" used there:

Developing Guest Excellence at Bradley Memorial

1. Convert the Organizational Culture.

- If you're not there yet, begin to develop a
  servant leadership style. Start it at the top
  and weave it throughout the organization.
- Paint the vision for the future for the
  organization. The CEO communicates it over
  and over in a multitude of ways to develop
  employee pride in the organization.
- Concentrate more on developing employee
  relationships; create opportunities for
  employees to interact frequently and
  consistently. Start with the senior staff. Follow
  Bradley's Tuesday morning meeting philosophy.
- Develop a "family" atmosphere in the
  organization. Encourage it in as many ways as
  possible within the management style. Tear
  down walls between departments and among
  all levels of management.

2. Sanction Employees to Serve.

- Bury administration. Knock down the walls.
  Develop an organizationwide management
  team. Encourage participative management.
  Hold annual management retreats.
- Treat employees as guests. Listen to them,
  develop their talents, pay them well, and give
  them opportunity to provide input to
  organizational decisions. Trust them but hold
  them accountable. Provide training and

educational opportunities. Empower them to act on their own and then back them up.

3. Focus on Customer Service.

(After Step 1 and 2 have begun and when the employees are more receptive to the idea.)

- Get employees together from a wide range of departments on a special task force (adding a consultant is optional, but in many situations it can be a big help). Create hundreds of ideas for improving patient satisfaction in your organization.

- Create your own customer service creed and promote it constantly.

- Reorient all employees to the emphasis of excellent customer service. Impress new employees with the organization's stance on customer service.

- Set up a reward system for employees for good customer service.

- Talk customer service up. Communicate it in as many ways as you can. Keep the interest keen within the organization.

- Get constant feedback from patients through surveys and focus groups. Follow up with specific action where indicated. Give employees feedback on how they are doing based on survey results.

- Train and educate all your employees on all aspects of customer service. Make it continuous, fun, and practical.

- Make patient relations issues part of all employees' salary reviews. Make it constitute as much as 25 percent of their performance score.

- Create an organizational mascot and use it in as many ways as possible.
- Form community groups from citizens around the hospital to help promote the hospital and the staff's commitment to excellent service. Seek their ideas.

12

CHAPTER

Guaranteed Service

Lake Forest Hospital's Approach to Customer Satisfaction

When we heard the term *guaranteed service* being applied to a healthcare setting, we were pretty skeptical. Candidly, we expected to see another well-intended customer relations "sensitivity" strategy: nice words, but little if any action. We weren't even sure we knew what *guaranteed service* meant.

That was before we met with Jim Killian, executive vice president at Lake Forest Hospital, a 250-bed facility in Lake Forest, Illinois, one of Chicago's most affluent suburbs. Killian outlined the facility's position:

> Like most hospitals that operate in this very competitive market, we are very concerned about what our patients think. About a quarter come from Lake Forest, another 30 percent come from the surrounding northern and western suburbs. The rest come from throughout the area. We take nothing for granted about our patient base—they have high expectations and no shortage of alternatives if we don't meet their needs.

First impressions can be deceiving, but as we walked around the facility, it quickly became apparent that this was not a "run-of-the-mill" hospital. As we stood in the main entrance, we were immediately impressed by its home-like atmosphere: gleaming floors, accented with green marble; rich-looking cherry furniture with solid fabric upholstery throughout the waiting rooms and community areas; patient rooms decorated with paintings and floral wallcoverings. The decor is simple, but elegant. But that doesn't fully describe what is unique about Lake Forest Hospital.

"I don't think bricks and mortar and a beautiful property have anything to do with it." Killian summed up what each of us had observed as we walked throughout the hospital. "It's really all about people." Clearly, our perception of the staff at Lake Forest was that they were every bit as unique as the attractive surroundings. We saw it in the way they greeted patients, responded to fellow workers, and accommodated visitors' requests.

Their promotional brochure makes the following bold commitment: "At Lake Forest Hospital . . . we will do whatever it takes to meet the needs of our customers and exceed their expectations." The staff promise their "customers" that they will be treated with respect, compassion, and caring. The guarantee goes on to state that staff will "respect your time, your privacy, your fears, and your need for information and reassurance."

EMPLOYEES EMPOWERED TO RESPOND

But the customer service commitment doesn't stop at a brochure. If someone reports that "their expectations" were not met, all employees who have received "guaranteed service" training are empowered to respond. Stated Killian:

> Employee empowerment is great, if you give them the education and the knowledge to use the empowerment

effectively. Our goal is to react appropriately if things have not gone as positively as we would hope. You can't just pass a wand over somebody's head and say "Thou shall be empowered"; they need to know how to identify the other person's true concerns.

The program was the brain child of CEO Bill Reis, who had always held to an overriding management philosophy of "guaranteed service." Killian reported:

> Bill applies the concept of "exceeding expectations" to every aspect of his life. As a result, the management staff of the hospital has adapted similar standards. A few years ago he suggested that "we make it more and more obvious to the public that we are willing to stand behind our service." Bill often reminds us that our employees provide Lake Forest with our "competitive edge."

According to Bill Reis, "Anyone can have a building, anyone can buy the equipment, but not everyone can have the employees and the customer service we provide here."

The facility's first attempt at formalizing the concept was a canned guest relations program called "Hospitality" initiated in 1986. It was largely a training program that focused on human relations skills—telephone answering, communication techniques, and other common courtesies. Ultimately, Lake Forest devoted six or seven trainers to expose their staff to human relations skills. But the skills training was just a foundation. Within a few years, the program evolved into the customized "guaranteed service" program, piloted in the day surgery unit in 1989.

Gail Okon, RN, P.A.C.U./day surgery unit manager, was one of the pioneers. "We drifted into it naturally," explained Okon. "Because we had an established tradition of quality care, it was not that big of a deal to guarantee it." The staff was consulted at the outset to ensure their commitment to the program. "We clearly expressed to all staff members that they would work collaboratively with the patient to decide what would be done to rectify an unsatisfactory situation." Kathy Conley, one of the unit's RNs, continues to be enthusiastic about the program. "I like the idea that when a situation arises, each one of us has the authority to do something to better it. I think it gives Lake Forest Hospital the edge over other healthcare institutions."

ANALYZED IMPACT

Before the program was taken hospitalwide in 1992, Lake Forest analyzed the impact on the facility.

- Of more than 3,100 annual day surgery cases, only 10 resulted in "guaranteed service" payouts.
- The percentage of credits to revenue was less than 0.0004 percent.
- Many patients use the program to voice concerns and refuse monetary compensation: "they just want to be heard."
- During the pilot, only two patients truly "abused" the program. Their comment upon a subsequent visit was, "What can I get this time?"

Okon summarized the analysis:

Once we began to talk about "guaranteed services" our thinking patterns changed, which influenced our behaviors. Our goal is no longer to meet expectations, but to exceed them. Lake Forest Hospital is a noncontentious atmosphere; we are all working together to ensure the best in patient care.

Interestingly, Okon's comment identifies one of the subtle dimensions of the "guaranteed service" program. On its own, it is only a "Band-Aid" for service problems. If all the employee does is react to the patient's complaint, no improvement is noted. Lake Forest uses the information gathered from guaranteed service payouts as input for its active CQI initiative. Jim Killian agreed: "Guaranteed service is a good tool to find out where you fall down, and when things don't go well, you have the ability to take immediate action for the patient. Unfortunately, if you don't fix the problem, if you're constantly apologizing for cold meals or late surgery schedules, you're not getting to the root of the problem. That led us into CQI as the next step."

The staff's reaction to the program is not exactly what Jim Killian expected:

> On its surface, the program didn't seem to threaten anybody. However, we needed to make sure that we could provide what we were guaranteeing, and that we could identify where we were coming up short. Predictably, there was some concern about the concept of employee accountability. We hadn't always done a good job of recognizing employee contributions—positive as well as negative. They simple weren't comfortable that we'd be any more successful this time. We thought that was valid, and as a result took extra steps to ensure we were responsible in our actions. On the other hand, they were also given the authority—from line employees to board members—to take care of a situation when it happened. We were empowering people for the very first time, and in some cases, managers were very threatened by that. I think some of the managers had a harder time than most of the general staff.

PHYSICIANS INITIALLY PANICKED BY PROGRAM

But managers weren't the only ones feeling threatened. Physicians were initially panicked by the program. They thought the focus was on medical outcomes, which obviously no one could control. As a result, even the promotional brochure carries the disclaimer that *"Because of the nature of illness, we cannot guarantee the results of your medical treatment."* But Killian immediately interjected that "we can guarantee that people would be treated in a courteous manner." Killian said, "We've had a couple of our larger practices adopt the same standards of service, and have actually asked to have their staff go through the same training program that we've done here."

TRAINING REQUIREMENTS

The training is impressive. Two distinct "tracks" (one for line employees and another for managers) have been developed. The employee workshop initially focuses on the conceptual aspect of quality service and customer needs. Staff are provided with key customer concerns, as well as factors that impact "perception" of quality. But the material is based on the realities of day-to-day experiences, requiring participants to identify "moments of truth" from a patient's point of view.

Time is spent on identifying internal and external customers. Although the patient is the primary focus, the needs and expectations of fellow employees, physicians, and other organizations are identified and analyzed. An assessment of current quality levels is made to provide a basis for "goal setting" and action planning.

Finally, skill-based training is provided in human relations techniques—problem solving, verbal and nonverbal communication, active listening, and dispute resolution.

The management program provides the same basic level of training provided in the employee track but combines it with an introductory "attitude adjustment." Managers are sensitized to the changing business paradigm of the healthcare industry, as well as specific information regarding the JCAHO's principles of quality improvement. Clearly, the objectives of the Guaranteed Service program, as well as the employee and management workshops, speak directly to the JCAHO's new standards for quality assessment and improvement (see box).

NEW JCAHO STANDARDS FOR QUALITY ASSESSMENT AND IMPROVEMENT

1. The organization's leaders set expectations, develop plans, and implement procedures to assess and improve the quality of the organization's governance, management, clinical, and support processes.

2. The leaders undertake education concerning the approach and method of continuous quality improvement.

3. The leaders set priorities for organizationwide quality improvement activities that are designed to improve patient outcomes.

4. The leaders allocate adequate resources for assessment and improvement of the organization's governance, managerial, clinical, and support processes through:

   a. The assignment of personnel, as needed, to participate in quality improvement activities.

   b. The provision of adequate time for personnel to participate in quality improvement activities.

   c. Information systems and appropriate data management processes to facilitate the collection, management, and analysis of data needed for quality improvement.

5. The leaders ensure that the organization staff are trained in assessing and improving processes that contribute to improved patient outcomes.

6. The leaders individually and jointly develop and participate in mechanisms to foster communication among individuals and among components of the organization, and to coordinate internal activities.

7. The leaders analyze and evaluate the effectiveness of their contributions to improving quality.

Jim Killian pointed out that a recent JCAHO accreditation survey—often a traumatic event for a hospital and its staff—actually presented an opportunity for the concepts of "guaranteed service" to be highlighted in an unconventional way:

> One of the "hero stories" involved our physicist for radiology and radiation oncology, who happened to be in labor the first day of the survey. The physician surveyor had a number of technical questions about radiation safety documentation that only she could answer. In true "guaranteed service spirit" she'd said, "Call me if you need me." So we did. In between cleansing breaths, she answered the surveyor's questions, and when everything was answered, she promptly had a healthy baby girl.

The JCAHO team was astounded by the staff's commitment to the organization, their fellow employees, and the patients.

EMPLOYEES GIVEN "HOW-TO"

Employees are provided with specific "how-tos" on fulfilling guaranteed service promises. The guidelines are straightforward:

- Out-of-pocket expenses are reimbursed through the normal employee expense reimbursement system. (Immediate reimbursement will be arranged if necessary.)
- Cash is available 24 hours a day from a nursing supervisor for immediate patient payouts.
- Flowers and other items are available from the gift shop—all that employees need to do is identify themselves and briefly describe the situation.
- The dietary supervisor provides guest trays and complimentary meal passes based on employee requests.

• Credits to patients' bills can be made directly from an employee's terminal.

Sound expensive? Killian reports that the program cost less than $10,000 last year and produced immeasurable patient and employee relations benefits.

But perhaps the best place to look for evidence of the program's effectiveness is through the patient's eyes. Lake Forest publishes a bimonthly newsletter called "The Record" that regularly reports examples of guaranteed service in action, and we reviewed some back issues. The newsletter's intent is to recognize and reinforce positive action. Here are some examples noted in the newsletter:

> An indigent patient was ready for discharge, but the unit nurse noticed that his clothes were badly soiled and tattered. Although she arranged to have the clothing repaired and laundered in the hospital's laundry, when two laundry employees saw the condition of the clothing, they decided that what the patient really needed was new clothes. They bought the patient new clothing out of their own pocket—the guaranteed service checkbook would have covered the expense, but the employees refused any reimbursement.

> Although delays are inevitable, an extended wait time caused an oncology patient significant discomfort. True to the instructions of the preadmission clerk, he'd left all valuables at home, including his wallet. When lunch time came and went, he felt pretty helpless. In the spirit of guaranteed service, the oncology secretary apologized for the delay and treated the patient to lunch in the coffee shop.

The hospital has collected several stories that illustrate guaranteed service in action. Senior management believes the program is nothing more than a formalization of what the staff do naturally. "But now they know we support their efforts and appreciate how it contributes to our unique atmosphere."

13

CQI and Patient Satisfaction

Irwin Press, cofounder of Press-Ganey, Inc., summarized it as well as anyone we talked to: "Patient survey data is meaningless unless you use it—and when you use it, you can truly make a difference." So we looked for a good example of a facility that took action based on the data they received in their patient surveys and found ourselves in Evansville, Indiana, at Deaconess Hospital, a 590-bed facility.

CQI EMPLOYED AT DEACONESS

Deaconess is an active participant in Press-Ganey's patient survey network and was recognized in 1994 for work it has done reducing noise levels on patient floors to minimize the disturbances to patients. Solutions included staff education and enclosing nurses' stations. Although the hospital is "still working on the problem," Deaconess claims early results are promising. We were actually more intrigued by the method used than by the results. Recent survey results have been mixed and candidly inclusive. But the hospital provides a textbook example of how CQI methods can be employed to investigate problem areas and identify potential solutions.

Deaconess jumped head first into the continuous quality improvement (CQI) wave of the early '90s. Their early initiatives included a number of site visits, as well as many hours of seminars and training. Joni Rahman, marketing analyst for the facility, told us, "We want to be one of the leaders in healthcare and we realize the methods and processes in place today may not be appropriate in the future. Change is a constant, and we are interested in any feedback that will help us to adapt to our patients' needs." During initial development, Deaconess created a CQI Task Force, a Quality Improvement Council, a quality coach position, and a quality improvement specialist position. The hospital's mission statement was rewritten to incorporate CQI. During the four years Deaconess has been actively involved in CQI, they have developed more than 20 Quality Advantage Teams (QATs). The noise level project was selected in the "second wave" of team creation.

ADDRESSING PATIENTS' COMPLAINTS ABOUT NOISE LEVEL

The hospital became concerned about excessive noise in June of 1992, when it found itself ranking in the 59th percentile for hospital noise levels. As a result, Deaconess established a problem statement for one of its CQI teams to "reduce the impact of noise level on nursing units as measured by patient satisfaction surveys."

FADE Process

The Noise Level QAT included members from administration, engineering, and maintenance, and used Organizational Dynamics, Inc., CQI process. ODI's approach consists of the *FADE* process: *focus, analyze, develop, and execute*. During each of these stages, the team achieves certain goals in order to continue to the next stage. An opportunity statement is developed in the *focus* stage; data is collected and analyzed in the *analyze* stage; a prospective solution is the result of the *develop* stage. Finally, during the *execute* stage, the solution is implemented and measured for improvement.

During the focus stage, the team brainstormed to generate a list of possible causes of excessive noise. With this information, a fishbone diagram was developed. This diagram was divided into four sections, each representing a different type of cause: people, method, material, and machines. To provide additional information, patient interviews were conducted, along with random observations of the nursing units.

A Pareto chart, which visually represents the distribution of occurrences being studied, identified

- Night shift activities
- Nurses stations
- Construction

as the top three sources of potential excessive noise.

During this early data collection phase, some "low-hanging fruit" opportunities (obvious, low-risk, high-impact, easy-to-implement changes) were identified to immediately reduce noise levels. On the list were repetitive weather announcements made over the hospital's public address system, noise generated from newspaper stands located throughout the hospital, and miscellaneous loud doors.

Multivoting, a CQI technique that helps to prioritize the team's position and potential actions, was used to identify three significant "opportunities for improvement": Employees at nurse's stations; patient visitation; and night noise. The team went on to develop an opportunity statement:

An improvement opportunity exists in reducing the noise level generated at the nurses station during the late evening and night time hours. This causes dissatisfaction among the patients as reflected on patient surveys. Reduction of the noise level should result in increased patient satisfaction.

As the team entered the analyze stage, additional data was collected from Press-Ganey patient satisfaction surveys. Surveys were correlated to specific nursing units, in order to determine nursing units with lowest scores. Three units were identified, and two were selected as test sites.

Input from Employees

Input was solicited from employees to help identify potential sources of excessive noise as well as to determine what they had been told by patients regarding noise levels. This phase concluded that the top five reasons for excessive noise were:

1. Talking and laughing by employees, visitors, and other patients.
2. Noise associated with shift changes.
3. Night shift nursing activities.
4. Evening shift nursing activities.
5. Day shift nursing activities.

With this information, the team entered the develop stage. Although a number of approaches were used to identify potential corrective action, the top three solutions ultimately determined through the multivoting process included:

1. Glass-in the nurse's station.
2. Use soundproofing materials/insulation on unit areas.
3. Provide headsets for patients.

Some additional ideas included using silent paging systems and employee awareness programs.

Once these solutions were discovered, additional data gathering occurred, and the team concluded that the noise cancellation technology associated with the second solution was cost prohibitive. The team once again multivoted and decided to proceed with glassing in the nursing station. The team used a number of approaches to gain buy-in and support from the staff, physicians, and administration. Ultimately, final approval was received, and construction began the execute stage in September of 1993.

The process took slightly more than 16 months. This is relatively fast by CQI standards but still painfully slow in terms of actual impact on patient satisfaction. Although the hospital did not disclose the cost of the initiative, any facility involved in its own CQI program is well aware of the investment of time and administrative support required just to complete the associated studies, surveys, and analysis. Deaconess concluded that the glassed-in nurse's stations were a positive way to reduce noise and protect patient confidentiality. However, the facility now has a hospital-wide reengineering initiative underway, and as a result has suspended further implementation of the team's recommendations.

The noise-reduction plan effectively illustrates our concern with this approach. The thoroughness associated with problem definition and methodical research associated with potential problem resolution are both its strongest asset and its weakest link.

The process simply takes too long. By the time you've identified the problem and implemented the solution, the problem may have changed. Or worse, the patient may have gone to your competitor.

14

CHAPTER

An "Aloha" Approach to Patient Relations

The Queen's Medical Center

Top-quality patient relations practices come in many different forms for the nation's hospitals, as you have seen in previous chapters. We saw another unique example of this at The Queen's Medical Center. Anyone entering The Queen's Medical Center (530 beds) in Honolulu, Hawaii, will notice immediately that something here is different. Patients are welcomed to the hospital by the scent of tropical flowers and the sound of ukeleles. Greeters meet the patients and provide valet service for their cars at no charge. Based on Hawaiian tradition, there's a strong influence of family. This creates the same kind of aloha you would feel in island hotels.

Lindsey Carry, director of the patient relations department, says the hospitalwide focus on patient relations is championed by the hospital's president, Arthur A. Ushijima. Carry says Ushijima and employees throughout the hospital consider quality patient relations to be a top goal of The Queen's Medical Center. The Queen's Medical Center has a unique background: It was founded by Hawaii's Queen Emma and King Kamehameha IV in 1859. Queen Emma went door-to-door soliciting funds to build an emergency clinic on the island, which had been devastated by several major epidemics that had wiped out a huge portion of the population. As a result, the hospital has a special mission of caring for all Hawaiians (and Pacific Islanders).

Measuring patient satisfaction is something that The Queen's Medical Center considers to be important. In many ways, the measurements have become a real science. The science is to do more, to go further in-depth and find out what patients really thought about their healthcare experiences, and to determine what issues are most important to patients. Originally, Carry told us The Queen's Medical Center used the Press-Ganey written surveys for its patients. She said they found them too mainland-oriented and not really geared to reflect the unique concerns of their patient population. Realizing the need to create a scientific survey that was right for them, Carry hired an outside research group, based in Hawaii, to help them work through the process.

SURVEYING FOR QUALITY INDICATORS

To begin revamping the survey process in April of 1994, the consulting group conducted eight hours of focus groups. The focus groups consisted of four different groups of 10 to 12 people who had recently been admitted as inpatients at The Queen's Medical Center. These groups were videotaped behind a one-way mirror, and staff members attended the sessions. From these focus groups, the consultants were able to identify 25 "quality indicators," or issues which the former patients deemed most important. From these 25 indicators, the consultants redirected their research to determine the 15 most important "quality indicators" among inpatient admissions.

A telephone poll was conducted with 450 discharged patients to validate the top 15 quality indicators. Then the patients were asked how well the hospital rated on each of the indicators during their last hospitalization. These results were then communicated to all levels of the organization. The quality indicators identified as most important to patients are as follows:

1. Care team is knowledgeable—patient feels he/she is in good hands.
2. Care team is well-informed about patients' medical condition.
3. Staff sensitive to patient's medical condition—makes him/her as comfortable as possible.
4. Staff respects patient's rights.
5. Patient and family informed about medical condition and treatment.
6. Staff treats patient professionally.
7. Patient feels he/she has say in decisions about his/her medical care and treatment.
8. Staff listens to patient.
9. Staff conveys warmth and friendliness.
10. Staff responds quickly to assistance requests.
11. Staff treats patient with compassion.
12. Patient is informed about self-care at home.
13. Staff shows respect for patient's privacy.
14. Staff gives patient encouragement and reassurance.
15. Staff anticipates patient's needs for comfort.

SET UP SPECIAL TEAM

The next step was to set up a "Performance Improvement Team" dedicated to improving patient satisfaction by setting up action plans based on the research. A 10-minute video called "What Our Patients Are Saying" was developed from the focus groups and is shown to all new hires, as well as to all ancillary department and nursing unit staff. After this process was completed, a new written survey was developed based on the quality indicators indicated as most important to their patients. The first part of the survey consists of 15 questions, asking respondents to rate their experiences on a scale of 1 to 10, 1 being strongly disagree and 10 being strongly agree. In keeping with The Queen's Medical Center's philosophy, the emphasis here is caring. For example, the survey asks patients to respond to such statements as: "My care team was knowledgeable, making me feel I was in good hands." "The staff was warm and friendly." "The staff was encouraging and reassuring."

The second part of the survey asks about overall satisfaction. Respondents are given five choices and asked to check the one that most fits their impression, from, "Queen's fell far short of my expectations," to the top choice, "Queen's far exceeded my expectations." The survey also asks two open-ended questions with space for a reply: "What aspect of your hospitalization at Queen's impressed you the most?" and "Please tell us if there are any areas where Queen's can improve."

Reflecting the overall trend in the healthcare world toward measuring medical outcomes as a factor in patient satisfaction, the third part of the survey asks for "other thoughts" regarding medical outcomes. Respondents are asked to check one of five responses, from "Very dissatisfied with my medical results," to "Very satisfied with my medical results." Next, patients are asked, "If you needed hospitalization again, would you return to Queen's?" And finally, patients are given the chance to give the name, unit, and comments of any special staff members they would like to acknowledge.

Just as important as the survey process itself was communication to hospital employees about patient satisfaction. Carry says all results of the survey process, that is, "What do patients want?" have been communicated to all levels of the organization. This means every employee of The Queen's Medical Center in theory should understand more about the patient population he/she serves. This, of course, sounds great. The question is, do employees really pay attention to things like a patient survey? Another equally valid question is this: What incentive do employees have to care about patient concerns?

The answers to those questions are usually found in continual sharing of information (survey results) and consistent communication from senior management on the issue of patient satisfaction. This, in turn, should then be championed by department managers and staff members themselves.

CUSTOMER SERVICE BECOMES CONTAGIOUS

So, is every employee at The Queen's Medical Center excited about the mission of improved patient relations? Probably not. But the emphasis put on the subject by hospital management is designed to capture the vast majority of employees. This, in turn, becomes contagious. As one staff member goes out of his/her way, it is noticed by other employees. When this is noticed by co-workers, it is much more likely to happen again with others. So when the hospital constantly talks about quality patient relations, it is setting up an environment where it is appropriate to go out of your way for patients.

The final piece of the puzzle to get employee buy-in on patient relations is the management environment itself. If employees think senior management is merely expressing platitudes, then there is a small chance the program will be successful. If, on the other hand, employees sense a genuine caring for patients, a solid patient relations program has a real chance. So senior management's role at The Queen's Medical Center is key. These managers set the overall tone. When hospital employees consistently experience evidence from management that patient relations is important, they get a signal that it is appropriate for them to take it seriously themselves. We saw an abundance of evidence of this when we were on-site at the medical center.

For example, when a patient looks lost, do staff go out of their way to help out? Or if staff are having a bad day, do they go out of their way to avoid letting the patient know about it? It's the little things that contribute to quality patient relations. Senior management's role at The Queen's Medical Center plays a major part in making it happen.

HOW THE PATIENT RELATIONS DEPARTMENT WORKS

According to Carry, one key aspect of "managing" patient relations is the patient relations department. Carry has a staff of nine in her department. Six are patient relations representatives including three volunteers. Two work on the off-island housing program and there is one administrative secretary. To promote use of the patient relations department, a Patient Visitation program was initiated. Patient relations representatives are assigned to nursing units and meet with newly admitted patients to proactively address any concerns.

A colorful, easy-to-read brochure highlights the Patients' Rights and Responsibilities. If the patient is not in the room when the representative visits, an attractive tent card, similar to those used in hotels, is left informing the patient whom to contact should there be a complaint. The in-house television channel also promotes patients' contacting the department regarding issues they feel need resolution. Carry says she encourages patients to complain or bring up issues to her department. "We can assist patients with issues ranging from patient rights to parking. Should they have any questions, concerns, or special needs, they are encouraged to call their patient representative."

Carry says this approach of asking patients to work with patient representatives is good business. "Malpractice lawsuits are less likely to happen. We like to deal with issues as they come up," says Carry. In fact, Carry says an *increase* in patient complaints may actually be a positive sign, meaning that the patient representatives are relating to more patients. It also means the design of the system is sound, because it funnels patients into the patient relations department.

Carry added that results for improving patient relations do not rest alone with the patient relations department; "results of patient satisfaction are communicated to all levels of the organization." She described how the patient relations assistant positions are key to controlling patient complaints. The organization setup is fairly simple:

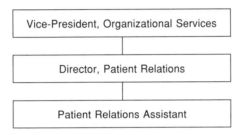

Carry said the primary contacts for the patient relations assistant are patients and their families, physicians, nurses, and clinical and nonclinical staff. The primary focus of the patient relations assistant is patient advocacy, problem resolution, and education. Carry also outlined the job description of the patient relations assistant, listing 11 of the major duties and responsibilities:

1. Identifies, assesses, and makes recommendations to director regarding situations in which preemptive intervention will result in reduced numbers of patient complaints and problems.

2. Informs patients, families, community, medical staff, administration, and employees on the role and function of patient relations as directed or required.

3. Provides counsel to patients and families regarding patient rights within the medical center.

4. Assists and participates in facilitating the grievance mechanism for patients exercising their rights; refers problems/concerns to appropriate staff and provides follow-up and advocacy for appropriate resolution under the direction of the director.

5. Assists patients with needs not routinely met in other medical center areas such as special parking rates, meal vouchers, VIP services, and so on.

6. Provides ongoing support and assistance to the patient relations volunteers as required.

7. Performs duties in a courteous and friendly manner that fosters superior customer service.

8. Participates in providing information on issues of patient rights, informal counsel, and community and hospital resources to the community, medical center, and medical staff.

9. Establishes and maintains working relationships with community health, welfare, and social agencies; maintains department resources on file.

10. Serves on committees and attends meetings as directed and required.

11. Maintains records and prepares statistics as required.

When you analyze the duties and responsibilities of the patient relations assistant, you will see that the position is designed to help patients with virtually any problem they may encounter.

One question you might ask in reviewing the duties of the patient relations assistant is, does it really work? And if it works, how do you know it? In this area, The Queen's Medical Center has done extensive research.

The patient relations department collects information regarding complaints for the following reasons:

- To maintain a comprehensive record of allegations, interventions, and resolutions of cases investigated.
- To determine patients' and families' needs and expectations.
- To identify trends throughout the medical center.
- To identify targets for performance improvement projects.
- To meet JCAHO and Department of Health standards.

The medical center also tracks complaint resolution. It breaks the complaint resolution into three categories:

1. Resolved.
2. Unresolved.
3. Unfounded.

One area of potential problems for the medical center is that often complaints are received and resolved directly by the departments receiving the complaint. Consequently, the statistics tracked by Queen's represent only those complaints received and investigated by the Patient Relations Department. Complaints are also categorized by area of concern. At Queen's there are nine major categories, illustrated in Table 14.1.

According to Carry, the extensive tracking of patient complaints helps The Queen's Medical Center better understand patients. Carry also told us about her role. She said her job has 10 major functions:

1. Formulation of department vision.
2. Ensuring that medical center staff support patient rights.

TABLE 14.1

Types of Complaints

Accessibility	Food	Physical Environment
• Received Inaccurate Information • Wait for Service	• Taste/Preparation/ Appearance • Correct Diet Plans	• Noise Level • Patient Unhappy with Room • QMC Property • Roommate Problems
Clinical Staff (Non-MD/RN) • Courtesy/ Communication • Efficiency/Service • Medical Care	**MD** • Courtesy/ Communication • Efficiency/Service • Medical Care	**Property** • Damaged • Misplaced • Stolen
Dissatisfied with Policies and Procedures • Billing Policy • Department Policy • Nonparticipation with Insurance • Queens Medical Center Policy	**Nonclinical Staff** • Courtesy/ Communication • Efficiency/Service • Patient Care	**RN** • Courtesy/ Communication • Efficiency/Service • Medical Care

3. Involvement in housewide performance improvement activities.

4. Resolution of patient and family complaints with emphasis on potentially litigious cases.

5. Inpatient and outpatient patient satisfaction projects:

  • Focus groups.

  • Telephone surveys.

  • Mail out surveys.

  • Quarterly and annual patient satisfaction reports.

- Analysis and trending of data.
- Patient satisfaction video.
- Patient satisfaction presentations throughout medical center.
6. Ensuring that JCAHO standards relative to patient rights are satisfied.
7. Strategic planning relative to healthcare reform.
   - Focus on outpatients/Pacific Rim.
8. Development of proactive patient-focused activities.
   - Patient visitation program.
   - Volunteer patient relations representative.
9. Collaboration with nursing in "transforming and enhancing the health paradigm."
10. Reporting on patient relations activities (compliments, complaints, and so on) to all levels of the organization.

These duties are all geared toward ensuring that the patient relations department runs smoothly and stays relevant into the future.

COMMITTED TO PATIENT RELATIONS

Our visit to The Queen's Medical Center showed a group of people committed to helping patients. Staff are also willing to track and measure results far beyond what average employees would do. As a result, they have put an effective program in place.

Entering The Queen's Medical Center and learning about its approach to patient relations, we had one initial reservation. Can accountability for patient relations rest with one department? In reality what we observed was something a little different. Although The Patient Relations Department is squarely in the middle of the effort to help patients, the overall program is much wider in scope. The entire medical center is tuned into the patient relations effort. This begins at employee orientation and continues with consistent feedback on the issue to all employees. So what we observed was an overall patient relations program that blends well with the unique patient population served by The Queen's Medical Center.

The program is geared to Hawaiians and Pacific Islanders, but the basic process staff are using could be emulated by any healthcare provider. First they have surveyed their patient population to find out just what is most important to their patients. Second, staff have assembled a process to proactively work with patients and resolve issues or problems as they come up. Finally, and probably most importantly, staff consistently "talk up" patient relations. This begins at the top of the organization and permeates the entire medical center.

So there is something different at The Queen's Medical Center. You'll notice it when you walk in the front door. But don't for a minute think this unique environment happens by chance. This environment is a result of well-planned action.

15
CHAPTER

Customer Service Commandos
Holy Cross Hospital's War to Improve Patient Satisfaction

Driving through this older, blue collar neighborhood on Chicago's south side it was a hard to envision it as the home of "the most improved" hospital in the history of Press-Ganey's patient satisfaction survey process. Holy Cross Hospital, a 346-bed facility, is located across the street from Chicago's infamous Marquette Park. Its functional-yet-austere appearance belies its national reputation for its commitment to total patient satisfaction. And their reputation is fast becoming "legend." They were named as the "large hospital" winner of *Hospital & Health Networks* Magazine's Fourth Annual Great Comebacks contest. They have eight active "commando teams" focusing on improving customer satisfaction at almost every conceivable level in their organization. During 1994–95, more than 60 hospitals have toured or consulted with the Holy Cross "Customer Service Commandos."

BACKGROUND OF HOSPITAL'S PATIENT
SATISFACTION EFFORTS

But candidly, it came as no surprise that it hasn't always been that way. There was nothing flashy or fake about this hospital. Holy Cross is not the obvious facility of choice for patients in a highly competitive healthcare market. Fourteen languages are spoken in the emergency department—definitely a diverse patient base. Yet, walking down the hallway, it has the feeling of a trip back to your home town: familiar, comfortable, and caring. Holy Cross has achieved a "customer-focused" environment that's not dependent on the physical surroundings of the facility. Many of the pictures on the walls are of satisfied patients: customers. That's not a bad touch, and a great calling card, in any market.

However, for five years, Holy Cross languished in the lower fifth percentile of Press-Ganey's patient satisfaction index. Liz Jazwiec, RN and "leader" of the emergency department at the hospital, has a practical view about the value of patient satisfaction.

> For us, it was a matter of survival. Our cash reserves had dwindled dangerously low over a very short period back in 1991, and our patient satisfaction survey scores were in the "cellar." We desperately needed to increase our market share and recruit primary care physicians. Candidly, its pretty tough to do those things under the best conditions, and if you're not providing patients with satisfactory service, it's all but impossible. We had to do whatever was necessary to improve our patient satisfaction scores.

Holy Cross implemented a number of stopgap financial measures to "stop the bleeding" in late 1991 and early 1992, with little measurable impact on patient satisfaction levels. They moved only 9 basis points, "peaking" at the fourteenth percentile. And they were frustrated. That's when Mark Clemons, CEO, and Quint Studer, senior vice president of strategic implementation, set a goal to be in the seventy-fifth percentile within 12 months. Studer explained the logic of the seemingly impossible 600 percent improvement goal. "Our intention was to be a 'premier' healthcare organization, and somehow patient satisfaction ratings in the fiftieth percentile just didn't say 'premier,' even though that would have been a significant stretch based on where we'd been. We really couldn't settle for less than the seventy-fifth percentile."

But why the focus on patient satisfaction when Holy Cross was still struggling financially? Clemons reasoned that low patient satisfaction scores were a symptom of more serious problems within his organization. "As a hospital, if patient satisfaction is not in your strategic vision, what are you there for? If you have a patient satisfaction problem, you have a problem with the values of the organization."

ADDRESSING PATIENT SATISFACTION WITH "SERVE"

Clemons explained that in his view the key to success in the quest for excellence was for the entire organization to gauge every action against the values the staff had adopted for the new Holy Cross Hospital: customer needs and expectations. Those values are service, excellence, respect, value, and enthusiasm (SERVE). "If an action is not actively contributing to our values, implementing a SERVE behavior, or adding value to a customer, we eliminate it," Clemons said.

As a result, organizational development is the centerpiece of Holy Cross' strategic plan. "Our employees have truly become our partners. We have an open book management style here. Our strategic plan goes out to all 1,500 'partners.' Each of the department leaders has both a yearly and 90-day work plan. If a leader is unable to improve patient satisfaction, we have to take action. Effort is no excuse for lack of results," Clemons stated.

Effecting the kind of fundamental organizational change apparent at Holy Cross required a revolutionary approach. Studer prefers the term "declaration of war." He felt denial was a real factor in their lack of success. "We didn't understand our scores, and many of our partners feared that disclosure of a problem could have a negative impact on their career. Just like any dysfunctional setting, we had to admit we had a problem before we could begin to 'heal.' Clearly, we had to change the corporate culture." He explained that the first major battle in their war to improve patient satisfaction was on "home turf."

> We looked inside and it wasn't pretty. We really didn't like who we were; what we had become. Our employee base, as well as our patient base, had become very diverse. We were treating drug addicts and trauma victims, and we didn't "like" them very much. We wanted badly to "blame" our problems on errors of our previous administration or on poor supervision. We somehow wanted to see ourselves as victims, because that would have made it easier to accept.

He paraphrased Stephen Covey. "Once we become a victim, we're no longer accountable for our own success or failure."

Studer feels this fundamental change in attitude, accepting responsibility for who they were, what they were to become, at every level of the organization, was the cornerstone of their successful turnaround. Within a very short time, he said, they started feeling good about themselves and the jobs they did. "Once we changed the culture internally, we were ready to take the war outside," he commented.

Commando Leaders

As the battle plan unfolded, it was clear that Studer's approach was not conventional. The "commando leaders" that were to become a key part of the new Holy Cross culture were asked to become responsible—accountable—for initiatives that would cross departmental boundaries, impacting areas for which they did not have direct control or supervisory responsibility. He explained that in his mind, true leadership in healthcare is achieved through facilitating change. He stressed that the interdependency of one manager on another ensured cooperation and ultimately the success of the whole plan, rather than the individual success of one department or manager. "Traditional organization structures don't provide a great deal of incentive for departments in a large institution to cooperate with one another. That's obviously counterproductive to our value of meeting the customer's needs rather than our own and had to be eliminated," Studer explained.

"Commando leaders" have the ability to "draft" troops from any department. As a result, some "partners" are actually participating in three or four of the eight commando teams or, as Quint Studer refers to them, "platoons."

The First Platoon: Customer Satisfaction

The first platoon deployed in the war to improve patient satisfaction at Holy Cross Hospital was charged with measuring customer satisfaction in all areas and improving satisfaction by coordinating measurement tools. Their first action was to eliminate all surveys except Press-Ganey. "We had to agree on one consistent measurement system. Departments had learned years ago that asking a question a different way could produce completely different results, so we had all kinds of surveys measuring the same thing. We were confused, the patient was confused, and we weren't improving," Studer stated.

Dan Dean, team supervisor of radiology at Holy Cross, was asked to become the "commando leader" of this initiative, and as result, has become the "guru of measurement" for many Press-Ganey participants. Liz Jazwiec, leader of the emergency department at Holy Cross, provided the accolades: "Dan can look at a Press-Ganey number and tell what you need to do to improve it. Not the obvious things; he can identify the subtle and, more importantly, effective actions that need to be taken. He's known throughout the industry and is contacted frequently by other hospitals."

Quint Studer provided an example the staff encountered with their physical therapy department. "Patient satisfaction scores for our PTs were very low and it didn't seem to make logical sense. From our observations, they were very friendly, consistently doing the things we felt were necessary to put a patient at ease. Dan helped us identify that the issue was not friendliness, but privacy. Many of the things that the staff were doing to be 'friendly' were conflicting with the patient's desire for privacy. We changed our approach, and our scores improved dramatically."

Dean also provided the hospital with a good reason to keep lengths of stay to a minimum. His research indicates that patient satisfaction scores decline significantly for patients whose length of stay exceeds five days.

Early in their efforts to improve, Dean realized that the conventional quarterly reporting of Press-Ganey was just too long to wait to determine whether a corrective action had affected a measurement successfully. He initially designed a system to provide monthly feedback and then decided that was too long. Weekly reports worked for a while, but now he is able to update his measurement database daily so that the commando teams have almost immediate feedback on customer satisfaction.

The Second Platoon: Customer Communication

The next platoon to be deployed focused on customer communication. Once again, the hospital felt that a conventional approach probably wouldn't produce the results they needed. They weren't particularly interested in changing brochures but did generate a patient admissions booklet and map as one of their early projects. According to Studer, the group's real objective was to communicate a positive message to a patient as early during his/her stay as possible:

> For a patient, the only really credible source that our customer satisfaction levels are high is another patient. It really doesn't matter what our brochures say or promise; if another patient relates a positive experience, it is far more likely that a patient will perceive our service positively. That's where the idea for the "Who's talking" campaign came from. We have pictures of satisfied patients saying good things about the hospital posted throughout the facility. We wanted patients to begin to see our best side as soon as possible: First impressions are critical.

One of the hospital's early failures ultimately became one of its greatest success stories. Studer jokes that the payer mix at Holy Cross is "government"—including a heavy influx of trauma patients from the emergency department. Staff currently have to be prepared to speak 14 different languages—and new Arabic dialects prevalent in the area are likely to add to the challenge.

The department had a history of low patient satisfaction scores and attributed its poor performance to the inherent challenges of an inner city ED. That was before Liz Jazwiec took over as commando leader for the team. She reported:

> We were in the eighth percentile, and dragging down the performance of the rest of the hospital. Most of the change was attitude, and I give Mark Clemons and Quint Studer most of the credit for changing the corporate culture. Once we took responsibility for our own success, we found we could be "winners." Last quarter we were in the ninety-eighth percentile.

Jazwiec's approach was broad based and included improving patient communication, minimizing wait times, and redesigning the facility. But she attributes most of the success to the attitude of the "partners."

The Third Platoon: Removing Patient Irritations

The next platoon was asked to "identify and remove patient irritations"—not an insignificant challenge. The team's initiative included addressing everything from the evaluation and improvement of parking accommodations to patient complaints about the billing and collection system. Food service, security, and the overall appearance of the facility received their attention.

But one initiative Jazwiec noted best summarized the "commando" touch, which differentiated even common types of patient satisfaction projects:

> We asked food service personnel to inquire about the patient's room temperature when they delivered meals. If the patient was concerned, the partner was instructed to go to the telephone immediately and request that the engineering department adjust the temperature. The building department handles the requests as a high priority. Patient response was phenomenal. They were surprised that they'd been asked; but when the employee took immediate action, many were astounded.

Other Teams

Other commando teams focused on areas that had been identified through the measurement process as having a significant impact on overall customer satisfaction:

- Physician satisfaction—Interestingly, Holy Cross physicians told the commandos that the number one thing the facility could do to improve their (the doctors') satisfaction was to better meet the needs of their patients. The hospital now provides physicians with a separate report of the satisfaction levels of each one's own patients. Together, 44 focus areas have improved since the team was organized. As a result, the hospital is successfully recruiting and retaining additional medical staff—a key corporate goal.

- Adding value—This team attempts to identify "little things" that add value to the patient's experience. As a result of the group's efforts, the hospital started providing free parking to outpatients and day surgery patients. They arranged to have "guest trays" available at the discretion of a partner; if a staff member feels it's appropriate, the tray is provided, no questions asked. The group's "tactical plan" calls for dozens of similar small, but significant initiatives to differentiate the Holy Cross experience.

- Setting standards of performance—To help determine the proper "standards" of partner behavior, the team asked for input from the customer-focus groups. Using their findings, the team defined a clear set of standards for attitudes and responses to call lights; partner appearance; phone etiquette; privacy; discharge planning; patient wait times; and other key customer service measurements. By clearly communicating the standards to the staff and rewarding staff who consistently exceeded expectations, the hospital was able to pinpoint areas to redress for an immediate impact on patient satisfaction scores.

- Linking human performance to customer need— Perhaps the quickest way to show corporate commitment to customer satisfaction is to effectively tie employee performance evaluation to customer feedback. This team was able to incorporate customer, peer, leader, and self-evaluation into the appraisal process. The objective is to *develop* employees, not add another level of judgment.

The result of the comprehensive program was a record turnaround in Press-Ganey performance. Holy Cross was in the lower thirteenth percentile in September of 1993;

they had improved their performance to the ninety-seventh percentile—a jump of 84 basis points, exceeding even their own most optimistic goals.

We were obviously impressed by the program but curious about whether the focus on customer satisfaction had paid off for Holy Cross financially. The slight but detectable smirk on Quint Studer's face told us he was ready for that question:

> Our inpatient admissions were up 5 percent this year, but perhaps more importantly, outpatient admissions were up 30 percent. Our cost per discharge was down markedly, from $4,400 to $4,100. We recruited 40 new physicians last year and have opened several new clinics. We went from being "unratable" two years ago to a BBB+ rating in our most recent $25 million dollar offering. Nobody is declaring victory, but we've won our share of battles.

Studer was anxious to add a closing comment. "As in every major undertaking in my life, I've learned a lot of lessons along the way. Perhaps clearest to me is that success has nothing to do with what you're doing for yourself. It's about what you do for others."

EPILOGUE

It's rather ironic to be saying providers of healthcare need to practice better customer service. (It's akin to saying church clergy should practice what they preach.) It also seems more than a little ironic that providers today often separate healing from compassion, communicating, friendliness, and a sincere concern for patients' emotions and feelings. Yet that's what thousands of former patients representing nearly half of the states reported during our 1995 research: There is a lack of caring and kindness by providers and a whole lot of indifference. Somewhere along the line, healing got separated from humanitarianism. Apathy replaced affability. Boorish behavior overcame benevolence and good nature.

The patients we surveyed and interviewed rated hospitals' customer service issues on average at a poor 7.7 on an index of 10, and physicians slightly better at 8.1. However, younger patients (under 35) rated their last hospital experience at a shabby 6.7 and physicians at a sorry 7.7. The younger generation is the work force. They are the ones to whom employers are listening, and they are the age group most dissatisfied with providers.

So it would seem this dispassionate indifference has created such impassioned hostility among its customers—patients—that they are rising up in a mock revolt. The managed care phenomenon has allowed for the public to rise up in mass and organize what one might call an insurrection against indifference.

And that undeniable insurrection will impact income to the providers, generally more or less of it depending how the provider reacts to the demands for better customer service. The provider who understands that will survive. The ones who do not, will not.

Patients passionately want a change in behavior by the staffs providing healthcare in this country. They justifiably want to be treated with dignity and decorum. They are not demanding the moon, just simple things like friendliness, a certain amount of compassion, and explanations of what is going on in their treatment and why. And, oh yes, patients detest waiting for hours for procedures that take minutes.

Our research reveals employers are moving swiftly toward making quality and patient satisfaction decisive issues. Managed care organizations will be their carriers of justice. And justice will be served. Customer service in the healthcare industry will become the new buzzword. Cost control is a given. How patients are treated is the new frontier.

Our findings also lead us to conclude that the vast majority of providers are not paying attention to the omens. Most don't hear the discontented masses forming outside their doors. They don't seem to sense the coming together of a disgruntled public and a willing majority of employers to create this crescendo of change.

But transform they must. Providers' penchant for putting customer service on a low priority will undergo a transformation in the next few years. The revolt has indeed begun; the providers are just a little slow to recognize the signs. But as revenue and patient volume are affected, the not-so-subtle message will echo loudly throughout the industry, and at long last the patient will certainly come first, foremost, and last.

Dave Zimmerman

I N D E X

Multihospital corporations, 99
Mystery patient, 69, 70, 76, 77,
    82, 89, 130–131, 136, 140,
    145–147

N

Networks, 38. *See* Health plan
Night shift activities, 179, 180
Noise level, 178–180
Noise level QAT, 178
Nonclinical staff, 189
Nonmanagement, 153
    employees, 156
Nonmedical staff, 63
Nonverbal communication, 172
Nurse manager, 158
Nurses, 77
    stations, 179, 180
Nursing, 193
Nursing director, 162
Nursing manager, 151–153
Nursing staff, 82, 153–155
Nursing station, 181
Nursing supervisors, 157–161,
    174
Nursing units, 178
    staff, 186

O

On-site surveys, 48
Organization structures, 199
Organizational culture, 154,
    163, 164
Organizational decisions, 164
Organizational management,
    115
Organizational mascot, 166
Organizationwide management,
    164
Out-of-pocket expenses, 174
    caps, 12

Outpatient patient satisfaction
    projects, 192
Outpatient procedures, 100
Outpatients, 193
Overcrowding, 84
Ownership, 156, 160

P

Paging systems. *See* Silent
    paging systems
Paradigms, 158. *See also* Health
    paradigm
Pareto chart, 179
Parking accommodations, 202
Participative management, 164
Partner appearance, 203
Patient accounts, 102
Patient admissions, 200
Patient base, 29
Patient care, 102
Patient centered care, 94–95
Patient collections, 92
Patient communication, 201
Patient complaints, 54, 96, 161,
    189, 192
Patient contact activities, 92
Patient dissatisfaction, 6–8, 75
Patient feedback, 2. *See also*
    Managed care companies
Patient focus groups, 92
Patient interviews, 6, 98
Patient irritations, 202
Patient needs, 88
Patient payouts, 174
Patient relations, 35, 163, 165,
    183, 188
    activities, 193
    aloha approach, 183–194
    assistant, 190
        positions, 189
    commitment, 193–194
    department, 188–193

nothing

S

Salary reviews, 165
Satisfaction index, 85
Self-confidence, 123, 124
Senior management, 154, 161, 175, 187, 188
  team, 156
Senior staff, 162
Sensitivity strategy, 167
Servant attitude, 163
Servant leadership, 117–135, 162, 164. *See also* Hospitals
Servant philosophy, 119
SERVE. *See* Service, excellence, respect, value, and enthusiasm
Service, excellence, respect, value, and enthusiasm (SERVE), 197–198
Services, 7, 63, 75
  industries, 85
  perception, 54–56
  quality, 32
  standard, 172
Service-oriented parameters, 17
SESCO employee opinion survey, 140
Silent paging systems, 181
Site facility, 125
Site visits, 178
Skill-based training, 172
Social agencies, 190
Socialization, 123
Spiritual conversion, 116
Staff, 185, 190
  buy-in, 99
  education, 177
  employees, 113
  friendliness, 60
  frustration, 84
  members, 187
  participation, 97
  training, 102, 103
Strategic plan, 197
Strategic planning, 193
Strategy, 14–16
Subscribers, satisfaction, 29
Summary reports, 49–50
Super department, 132–133
Survey data, 96
Survey format, 45–46
  questions, 46–47
Survey information, 20
Survey methods, 47–49
Survey process, 186
Survey programs, 95
Survey questions, 46
Survey results, 32, 56–62, 177
Surveys, 98, 199

T

Tactical plan, 203
Task forces, 132, 138, 163, 165
Team building, 146
  skills, 98
Team members, 141
Team-building, 131
  attitude, 130
Teamwork, 94
Technicians, 77, 80, 141. *See also* EKG technicians
Telephone answering, 169
Telephone assessment tools, 92
Telephone interviews, 48
Telephone surveys, 48, 92, 192
Time frames, 145–147
Timing, 47–49
Total quality management (TQM), 90, 129, 131, 132
TQM. *See* Total quality management
Training program, 112
Training requirements, 172–174
Treatment plan, 78
Trending reports, 49–50
Triage, 110, 114

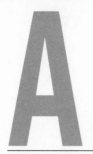

ABOUT THE AUTHORS

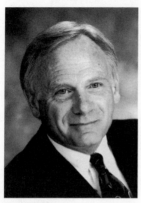

David Zimmerman

David Zimmerman has had 30 years of experience in the healthcare industry, including stints at Blue Cross and the HealthCare Financial Management Association, as well as 17 years in a variety of hospital management positions. He has made his mark as both an entrepreneur and an author.

For the past ten years, as President of his own healthcare consulting group, Zimmerman & Associates in Milwaukee, Wisconsin, David Zimmerman has helped hundreds of healthcare institutions throughout the country implement proven strategies for increased profitability. He is also the author of nine diverse healthcare books,

including this present effort, *The Healthcare Customer Service Revolution,* co-authored with his wife, Peggy, and Charles Lund. One of his previous books, *Reengineer-ing Health Care,* co-authored with John J. Skalko, was one of the most popular books in the industry in 1995; another book, *Cash Is King,* won him wide critical acclaim in the industry.

A popular nationally known lecturer, Mr. Zimmerman is quoted regularly in a wide variety of newsletters and national trade magazines, including *Hospitals and Health Networks* and *Modern Healthcare,* and has been interviewed numerous times on television and radio.

Peggy Zimmerman, prior to her present position as Executive Vice President of Zimmerman & Associates, held a variety of positions in the public relations and human resources departments of Miller Brewing Company, Blue Shield, and the Medical Society of Milwaukee County.

She lectures, presents seminars, and is active as a volunteer

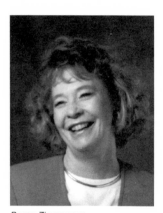

Peggy Zimmerman

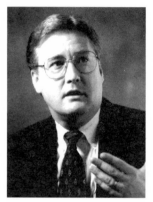

Charles Lund

for private organizations such as schools, churches, nursing homes, and Children's Hospital of Milwaukee. She has also organized and led a leadership program for teenage girls. In addition to being a wife and mother, she has also found time to assist in fund-raising activities for the Wisconsin Institute for Studies and Development.

Charles Lund, Vice President for Zimmerman & Associates, has an extensive background in hospital receivables consulting in addition to banking and charge-card collections. His financial background includes an assignment as Assistant Vice President of the Federal Reserve Bank of Chicago, where he managed the largest

check-processing operation in the world. He has directed the turnaround of three troubled bank operations, resulting in dramatic improvements in employee productivity and reductions in operating expenses. As an officer of the Federal Reserve, he presented a number of seminars to banking professionals.

In the healthcare field, he has worked as project manager for numerous diagnostic reviews, as well as serving as the on-site facilities manager for a number of the firm's turnaround assignments. He is also a popular seminar leader and has made numerous presentations at HFMA and AGPAM meetings.

Other books of interest to you from Irwin Professional Publishing . . .

THE FOR-PROFIT HEALTHCARE REVOLUTION
The Growing Impact of Investor-Owned Health Systems
Sandy Lutz and E. Preston Gee
ISBN: 1-55738-650-1

NOT WHAT THE DOCTOR ORDERED
Reinventing Medical Care in America
Jeffrey C. Bauer
ISBN: 1-55738-620-X

THRIVING ON REFORM
Meeting Tomorrow's Healthcare Challenges Today
E. Preston Gee
ISBN: 1-55738-618-8

STRATEGIC HEALTHCARE MANAGEMENT
Applying the Lessons of Today's Top Management Experts to the Business of Managed Care
Ira Studin
ISBN: 1-55738-631-5

HEALTHCARE MARKETING IN TRANSITION
Practical Answers to Pressing Questions
Terrence J. Rynne
ISBN: 1-55738-635-8

(Continued)

WORKING TOGETHER
Building Integrated Healthcare Organizations through Improved Executive/Physician Collaboration
Seth Allcorn
ISBN: 1-55738-614-5

Available in fine bookstores and libraries everywhere.

Lexington College

310 S. Peoria St. Ste. 512
Chicago, Il 60607 3534

Phone 312-226-6294
Fax 312-226-6405